Survival Skills In Trauma and Orth Surgery

Ben Marson ACF ST3 East Midlands North Rotation

Alex Dodds Consultant in Trauma and Orthopaedic Surgery,

Gloucestershire Hospitals NHS Foundation Trust

© 2016 MD+ Publishing

All rights reserved. No part of this publication may be reproduced, stored in a retrieval system or transmitted in any form or by any means, electronic, mechanical, photocopying, recording or otherwise without the prior permission of the publisher or in accordance with the provisions of the Copyright, Designs and Patents Act 1988 or under the terms of any licence permitting limited copying issued by the Copyright Licensing Agency.

Published by: MD+ Publishing

Cover Design: Alexander Logan

ISBN-10: 0993113850

ISBN-13: 978-0993113857

Printed in the United Kingdom

A catalogue record for this book is available from the British Library

Knowledge and best practice in this field are constantly changing. As new research and experience broaden our understanding, changes in research methods, professional practices, or medical treatment may become necessary.

Practitioners and researchers must always rely on their own experience and knowledge in evaluating and using any information, methods, compounds, or experiments described herein. In using such information or methods they should be mindful of their own safety and the safety of others, including parties for whom they have a professional responsibility.

With respect to any drug or pharmaceutical products identified, readers are advised to check the most current information provided (i) on procedures featured or (ii) by the manufacturer of each product to be administered, to verify the recommended dose or formula, the method and duration of administration, and contraindications. It is the responsibility of practitioners, relying on their own experience and knowledge of their patients, to make diagnoses, to determine dosages and the best treatment for each individual patient, and to take all appropriate safety precautions.

To the fullest extent of the law, neither the Publisher nor the authors, contributors, or editors, assume any liability for any injury and/or damage to persons or property as a matter of products liability, negligence or otherwise, or from any use or operation of any methods, products, instructions, or ideas contained in the material herein.

Images
Figures 1.2 and 1.3 kindly reproduced with permission from OpenStax College
Figure 5.1a kindly reproduced with permission from Wellcome Library, London
Figure 9.0 kindly reproduced with permission from Centers for Disease Control and Prevention, National Center for Health Statistics

Preface

Like many ventures, this book was conceived as a discussion between friends at a deanery social. The premise was simple, we identified that life as an Orthopaedic SHO is not straightforward, especially in the first few months of a rotation. As Orthopaedics is a massively postgraduate speciality, with little coverage of the subject in international medical school curricula, new trainees need as much help as they can get. Topics and skills will be new and unfamiliar, and the working team structure is very different to that in other specialities.

We knew that a guide to getting a foot hold in that first Orthopaedic job would have made our lives easier and more enjoyable. Taking the on-call bleep for the first time is daunting, and a reference for the management of common conditions and referrals from ED and other specialities was planned. Importantly, the way ward cover is provided is changing with more hospitals using hospital at night or cross-cover schemes. This book is also for anyone who is required to cover Orthopaedics by night, to help in those moments when you are unsure if you should call for help from the registrar.

Each chapter begins with a checklist to aid you in your initial approach and covers the most important orthopaedic emergencies and management options.

This book has been a team effort, and I am indebted to Adrian Brennan for acting as a soundboard for initial ideas, to Alex Young for his patience in waiting for drafts of the manuscript and tireless organisation and formatting. Thank you Lisa Wallis, for putting up with annual leave spent at the computer and for checking every word before publication.

Ben Marson

CONTENTS

Introduction 4
    0.1 Finding support 6
    0.2 Ward duties 6
    0.3 Learning opportunities 7
    0.4 Transferable skills 7
    0.5 Suggested curriculum. 8

Chapter 1: Orthopaedic Basic Science 12
    1.1 Bone healing 14
    1.2 Pre-op planning 18
    1.3 Methods of fixation 18

Chapter 2: The Trauma Call 22
    2.1 An introduction 25
    2.2 Preparation. 25
    2.3 Primary survey 26
    2.4 Secondary survey 27
    2.5 Damage control 30

Chapter 3: Upper Limb Injuries 34
    3.1 Distal radius fractures. 38
    3.2 Forearm fractures 40
    3.3 Elbow fractures 41
    3.4 Humerus fractures 42
    3.5 Dislocated shoulder 44
    3.6 Other presentations 46

Chapter 4: Hand Injuries 52
    4.1 Metacarpal fractures 55
    4.2 Carpal bone fractures. 58
    4.3 Nail bed injury. 60
    4.4 Tendon injuries 60
    4.5 Flexor sheath infections 61
    4.6 Other presentations 62

Chapter 5: Lower Limb Injuries 66
    5.1 Femoral fractures 69
    5.2 Knee injuries 70
    5.3 Tibial plateau fractures 75
    5.4 Tibial shaft fractures 76
    5.5 Ankle fractures 77
    5.6 Other presentations 79

CONTENTS

Chapter 6: Infection **84**
   6.1 Cellulitis 87
   6.2 Osteomyelitis 88
   6.3 Septic arthritis 90
   6.4 Bursitis 91
   6.5 Periprosthetic infection 92

Chapter 7: Spines **96**
   7.1 Back pain 100
   7.2 Cauda Equina syndrome 101
   7.3 Discitis and psoas abscess 102
   7.4 Spinal fractures 104
   7.5 Cervical myelopathy 106
   7.6 Other presentations 107

Chapter 8: Hip Fractures **108**
   8.1 Intracapsular fractures 112
   8.2 Extracapsular fractures 113
   8.3 Subtrochanteric fractures 114
   8.4 Pathological fractures 115
   8.5 Other presentations 116

Chapter 9: Paediatrics **120**
   9.1 Supracondylar fractures 123
   9.2 The limping child 125
   9.3 Growth plate injuries 128
   9.4 Femoral fractures 129
   9.5 Non-accidental injury 130
   9.6 Other presentations 131

Chapter 10: Elective Surgery **136**
   10.1 Total hip replacement 139
   10.2 Total knee replacement 142
   10.3 Arthroscopy 143
   10.4 Post-Op: AKI 144
   10.5 Post-Op: hyponatraemia 146

Chapter 11: Next Steps: A Career In Orthopaedics **148**
   11.1 Training scheme overview 148
   11.2 Work-based assessments 150
   11.3 Courses and qualifications 154
   11.4 Audit ideas 154
   11.5 Interviews 156

Introduction to Trauma and Orthopaedic Surgery

How To Get The Most Out Of Your Time

Introductory Chapter Contents

1. Finding support	p6	4. Transferable skills	p7
2. Ward duties	p6	5. Suggested curriculum	p8
3. Learning opportunities	p7		

3 Topics Not To Miss

1. Manipulation of a fracture
2. Aspiration of a joint
3. Assist in a joint replacement

Welcome to your rotation in orthopaedics. This book is written with foundation trainees in mind, but is equally applicable for medical students, early years trainees and core surgical trainees entering a rotation in trauma and orthopaedics.

As an overview, the foundation programme was developed in 2005. Graduating medical students are enrolled into a two-year Foundation Programme. This programme is designed to prepare new doctors first for full registration with the General Medical Council (GMC) and then for application and entry into specialist training.

In 2014-2015, approximately 30% of the South West Foundation trainees had a four month rotation in Trauma and Orthopaedics as part of their FY2 year. While it is anticipated that some of these trainees will be inspired to follow a career into Trauma and Orthopaedics via Core Surgical Training, it is understood that most of the FY2 doctors will choose alternative careers in GP, A&E, acute medicine or other specialities. This book has been designed to maximise transferable skills and knowledge to prepare trainees to understand the assessment of orthopaedic patients in a wide range of settings. Most importantly, it will flag up key orthopaedic emergencies – those which are severe enough to require immediate action, even if this involves waking the registrar in the middle of the night.

This book will act as a guide for common presentation and situations. It has been written by a team who have all survived (and remember) holding the SHO bleep and being the first on during an on call or night shift. The presentations have all been selected as they cover common referrals from the Emergency Department and GPs. While this book will increase your confidence, it does not remove the need for common sense. If you see something that concerns you, or you are not sure what to do then do not hesitate to call your senior, the registrar or consultant. They would much rather be called and asked than a patient come to harm.

Introduction to Orthopaedics

Things to do:

- Aspirate a knee
- Reduce a shoulder
- Apply a plaster
- Manipulate a wrist
- Close a wound

Things to see:

Theatre

- Total hip replacement
- Total knee replacement
- Knee arthroscopy
- Dynamic hip screw
- Hemiarthroplasty
- Cephlomedullary nail for femoral fracture

Clinic

- Knee clinic
- Shoulder clinic
- Paediatric clinic
- Plaster room
- Ortho-geriatric / falls clinic

Things to consider:

Your personal goals

- Do you need more time in theatre or clinic?
- Are there specific procedures you want to see?

Negotiate time off the ward

- Who will cover you?
- How will you repay them?

Other objectives

- Audit/ research
- Teaching
- Courses

A* ORTHOPAEDICS

Surviving a trauma meeting is much easier with a system for presenting x-rays.

1. Patient's name and date of birth
2. Describe the view taken (PA/AP/oblique/lateral)
3. Is there a fracture?
4. Is it open (may not be apparent)?
5. What bone is broken?
6. What part of the bone is broken? (Diaphysis/shaft, proximal/distal 1/3, intra-articular)
7. Are the fragments disconnected? (displaced)
8. Is it in joint? (dislocated)

Introduction

1. The problem with orthopaedics: where is the support?

For many years, orthopaedics has had a problem with its image as a training rotation. Everyone is busy, with the consultants and registrars tied up in elective and fracture clinics or in theatre doing lists. For some, the elective operating may not occur in the same hospital as the trauma work and there is a lot of sharing of the junior members of staff with a loss of the traditional team structure.

This creates a problem and a disconnection between trainees and trainers. Foundation trainees often complain about a lack of supervision while working on the wards and while on call. With ward based systems of working this can feel even worse but you are not alone. There is support available but unfortunately the registrars and consultants are unlikely to perform ward rounds in the same format as our medical colleagues. However, if you feel you cannot get help on an orthopaedic issue, there are various sources of help that you can use:

1. **The team registrar or consultant.**
At the beginning of your placement make friends with the departmental secretaries and get a copy of the consultants' job plans. This will give you a good idea as to where to look first. A telephone call is a good way to get quick advice, but if you can go and talk directly with the senior please do. If this means getting changed into scrubs or going and talking in clinic then great. It will give you a chance to present a history and plan and get teaching around the decision making and build your confidence for the future.

2. **Registrar on call**
Again, they will often be in theatre (often lead lined, so don't rely on mobile telephone signal) or clinic.

3. **Fracture clinic**
There will be seniors working most days in fracture clinic who can be approached for advice. They will be able to provide a solution, or at least direct you as who best to ask to solve your questions.

2. The ward duties

Depending on your unit, daily duties will differ. However, common themes include:

1. **Ward round**
a. Every patient needs to be seen by a medical practitioner every day with clear documentation in the notes.

b. Most patients should be recovering from injury, theatre or awaiting investigations so a simple screening tool may be used:

i. Review reason for admission
ii. Patient well / unwell
iii. Review observations, urine output and recent blood tests
iv. Check wound(s)
v. Check calves soft
vi. Confirm mobilisation status (full, partial or non-weight bearing) and progress with physiotherapy
vii. Consider discharge planning

2. **Paperwork**
a. Patients who have had major surgery (joint replacement, fixation of neck of femur fractures, intramedullary nails) will require postoperative bloods including a haemoglobin and urea and electrolytes

b. Request x-rays for patient with new metalwork that have not been imaged in theatre (e.g. joint replacement)

c. Prepare discharge summaries. This seems to be getting ever more time consuming and is being prioritised by nursing and managerial staff as bed numbers are contracting and as early discharge is being promoted.

3. **Other jobs (depending on hospital)**
a. Preparing cases for mortality and

morbidity (often forgotten until a week before presentation, try and be organised and collect as you go)

b. Audits – aim to complete at least 1 closed loop audit per year

c. Pre-assessment – usually structured, you may be required to do a pre-assessment proforma or just review ECGs to prevent patients being cancelled on the day of surgery.

3. Learning opportunities

With this hefty list of jobs, it may seem impossible to gain experience in orthopaedics. For this, you will need to work together with your fellow SHOs and rota coordinator. Work out when you are likely to be less busy or find time to be released from the wards to attend clinic or theatre.

It may feel un-exciting, but theatre is a great place to interact with the consultants and learn more technical skills as well as the interesting aspects of joint replacement and trauma management. If you don't make it to theatre then the consultants will struggle to teach you, as your paths will not overlap on a regular basis. The best places to learn are:

- Theatre
- Fracture clinic
- Elective clinic
- Plaster room
- Emergency department
- Ortho-geriatric / anaesthetic / pre-assessment clinic

Negotiate hard and find ways of getting these opportunities and you will learn and get so much more out of the rotation than being stuck on the ward filling out discharge summaries for 4-6 months.

During the rotation, you should aim to learn how to perform:

1. Aspiration of knee joint
2. Reduction of distal radius fracture under haematoma or Bier's block
3. Application of backslab
4. Remove a full cast (Plaster of Paris or Polymer)
5. Closed reduction of dislocated shoulder
6. Scrub and assist in arthroplasty surgery
7. Interrupted or subcuticular wound closure

If you are not getting these opportunities then speak to your registrar or your educational supervisor.

4. Transferrable Skills

We know that while 30% of foundation doctors will do orthopaedics we will not convince everyone to be future surgeons. However, the skills that you can learn outside of the ward will make your placement more enjoyable and more useful whatever your chosen career destination. Remember, musculoskeletal medicine appears in most specialities as it is such a broad system, and with comorbidities you will see "orthopaedic" patients in your future practice. You don't want to be the GP who misses a septic arthritis or the medical SHO who can't suture a scalp laceration when the patient slips on the ward.

Suggested learning opportunities for different career destinations are listed below. Common themes are enhancing your basic surgical or interventional skills, audit, and patient assessment skills. Communication and team working are also common skills that you will be developing, especially if you are working together to get additional educational opportunities.

5. Suggested curriculum

On completion of a four month rotation, FY2 doctors should be expected to have an understanding of the pathology, diagnosis and management of the following conditions: (topics with a * have been identified as priorities for the National Undergraduate Curriculum from the Royal College of Surgeons of England – these would make good talks to teach your local medical students).

	Trauma
Ankle fractures	i. Weber classification ii. Identification of talar shift iii. Reduction of displaced fracture iv. Indications for operative management
Proximal femoral fractures*	i. Classification of fractures ii. Management strategy – fixation vs excision arthroplasty
Cervical spine fractures	i. Application of in-line stabilisation / triple immobilisation ii. Indications for imaging iii. Interpretation of c-spine radiographs
Proximal humeral and shoulder fractures	i. Ability to identify proximal humeral + clavicle fractures ii. Understand methods of conservative management iii. Understand indications for surgery
Wrist fractures	i. Identify Colles' type, Smiths and Volar Barton fracture ii. Method of reducing fracture iii. Able to identify unstable fracture pattern
Pelvis fractures and polytrauma*	i. Mechanisms of injury ii. ATLS protocol iii. Management of open fractures
Compartment Syndrome	i. Risk factors and Diagnosis ii. Investigations (normal compartment pressures) iii. Management

Non-trauma

Septic arthritis*	i. Assessment and investigation ii. Kocher's criteria iii. Management
Osteomyelitis	i. Typical causative agents ii. Imaging iii. Principles of conservative and operative management
The limping child*	i. Potential cause by age ii. Imaging iii. Management
Cauda equina syndrome*	i. Typical history ii. Examination findings iii. Management options
Hip and knee osteoarthritis	i. Examination findings ii. Imaging iii. Management options (TKR vs Uni, THR vs resurfacing vs Metal on Metal)

Clinical Governance

Audit	i. Understand the principles of audit ii. Be involved in an audit cycle of an orthopaedic issue and present to peers

Introduction

Educational opportunities to help with other careers during your orthopaedic rotation

Acute Medicine	• Ward round assessment of patients • Electrolyte and fluid balance • Ortho-geriatric assessment of patients and falls clinics
Anaesthetics	• Peri-operative management of patients • Hands on technical skills • Situational awareness in trauma calls
Clinical Oncology	• Oncology MDTs • Management of pathological fractures • Calcium balance in post-operative patients • Breaking bad news (neck of femur fractures)
Clinical Radiology	• Trauma meetings • Musculoskeletal imaging • CT guided biopsy for infection or tumour
Combined Infection Training	• Managing orthopaedic infections • Infection and revision surgery MDTs
Emergency Medicine	• Trauma • Trauma • Trauma • Manipulation skills • Clinical decision making while on-call
General Practice	• Identification of orthopaedic emergencies • Aspiration and injection of joints • Basic surgical skills

Introduction to Orthopaedics: Educational Opportunities

General Surgery	• Basic surgical skills • Anatomy • Managing peri-operative patients
Neurology and Neurosurgery	• Assessment and management of spinal patients • Identifying cauda equina syndrome • Neurological exam in spinal clinics
Oral and Maxillofacial Surgery	• Understanding of fracture fixation • Basic surgical skills
Paediatrics	• Communication with parents and children • Non accidental injuries • Multi-disciplinary working
Plastic Surgery	• Basic surgical skills • Burns • Hand clinic and lists
Psychiatry	• Complex needs on the trauma and Ortho-geriatric wards • Anxiety, depression and self-harm • Risk assessments
Rheumatology	• Joint injection in knee clinic • Management of gout and septic arthritis • Joint replacement in rheumatoid and psoriatic arthritis

Chapter 1

Chapter 1: The Basic Science of Trauma and Orthopaedic Surgery

How To Look Like An Expert In The Trauma Meeting

SCIENCE

Chapter 1: Basic Science Contents			
1. Basic sciences of bone healing	p14	b. Plates	p19
2. Pre-op planning	p18	c. External fixators	p20
3. Methods of fixation	p18	d. Intramedullary nails	p20
a. Lag screw	p19	e. Tension band wires	p21

Introduction

Principles of fracture fixation underpin all emergency orthopaedic operations from intramedullary nailing to external fixation, be it in the little finger or femoral shaft. Understanding these principles is vital to appreciate the decision making process for selecting different modes of fixation and for planning operations when it is your turn to take responsibility.

This chapter provides an overview of fracture fixation to give an early-years trainee an adequate footing to understand fixation techniques. Further, more detailed courses are available and are vital when a trainee is ready to progress from basic to more advanced understanding of these techniques.

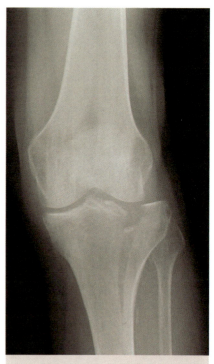

Lateral tibial plateau fracture

12

Fracture fixation checklist - Part 1: Fractures

Which Bone?	• Upper or lower limb? • Isolated injury or multiple injuries? • Is that bone essential for function, e.g. forearm in a person who uses crutches? • Open / closed? • Neurovascular status?
Where in the Bone?	• Shaft? • Intra articular?
What do you need to achieve?	• Primary bone healing with cutting cones? or • Secondary bone healing with callus?
What are the patient factors?	• Bone quality • Medical issues • Life expectancy • Compliance

Fracture fixation checklist - Part 2: Fixation

Primary bone healing	• Anatomical reduction • Restore anatomy, joint lines and normal function • Rigid fixation e.g. forearm fractures or ankle fractures
Secondary bone healing	• "Social" reduction (restore axis, length and rotation) • Hold long enough for the bones to heal • Healing with callus • Relative stability e.g. external fixator, IM nail, plaster cast

Chapter 1

1. Bone Healing

Though the understanding of the mechanism of bone healing may appear less practical than the other topics in this chapter, it is actually the most important knowledge for a trainee to grasp when dealing with fixing fractures.

A bone is a living structure. It is dynamic and reacts to its environment. Its structure is unique in the body with several cell types regulating bone formation and resorption (Figure 1.1). The three cell types are osteoblasts, osteoclasts and osteocytes. Osteoblasts are undifferentiated mesenchymal stem cells and produce osteoid (unmineralised bone). Osteoclasts are cells which have originated as macrophages and monocytes and have been stimulated to produce multi-nucleated osteoclasts. These are the only cells with the ability to resorb bone. Finally, the osteocytes are osteoblasts that have become entrapped by calcified bone matrix.

In addition to its cellular components, the strength of bone is derived from the extracellular matrix. This matrix is divided into inorganic and organic components, with differing properties. The inorganic component is mainly Calcium hydroxyapatite. This forms 60% of a bone's mass and is strong in compression. The organic component is Type 1 collagen which is strong in tension. Calcium hydroxyapatite resists compression better than collagen resists tension, so bone fails by distraction as the collagen fibres fail.

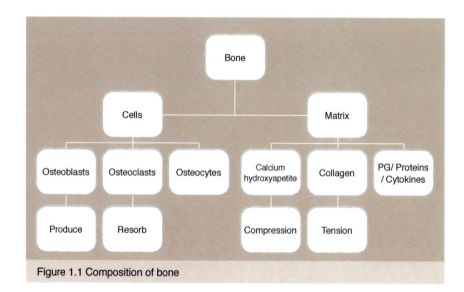

Figure 1.1 Composition of bone

Blood supply

Protection of the blood supply to a bone is vital in order to prevent bony necrosis and failure of union. Selection of fixation method will be determined to preserve as many of the following nutrient supplies to the bone (Figure 1.2):

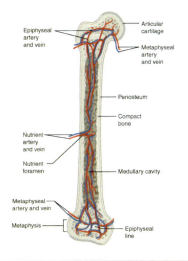

Figure 1.2 Bone blood supply

1. The diaphyseal nutrient artery: This is the most important supply of arterial blood to a long bone. One or 2 principal diaphyseal nutrient arteries first pass obliquely through the cortical bone. These arteries then divide into ascending and descending branches and supply the inner two thirds of the cortex and medullary cavity.

2. Metaphyseal and epiphyseal arteries: Numerous metaphyseal and epiphyseal arteries supply the ends of bones. These blood vessels mainly arise from the arteries that supply the adjacent joint.

3. Periosteal arterioles: Several of these vessels supply the outer layers of cortical bone.

The blood flow around a bone is usually inside out (centrifugal) with lots of anastomotic connections. If the endosteal supply is damaged then the periosteal supply is able to increase and take over. If this occurs then the flow is reversed (centripaedal). This is the method for preserving and increasing the blood supply when reaming for placement of an intramedullary nail.

Fracture healing

Fractures heal either by primary or secondary bone healing. Each of these has specific advantages and disadvantages, and the mode is selected by the configuration and stability of the fracture.

Primary bone healing

Primary bone healing occurs with cutting cones healing bone ends that are in close proximity. Osteoclasts are involved in forming these cutting cones. These tunnel across the fracture site when there is contact between bone ends or a minute gap between fracture ends. This cutting cone leaves a path for blood vessels and osteoblasts to follow, laying down lamellar bone in form of new osteons.

In order for primary bone healing to occur there must be no motion between the fracture surfaces under functional load. This is absolute stability. Primary bone healing is very intolerant of strain and movement at the fracture site. Alongside absolute stability, anatomic reduction and compression are required to encourage primary bone healing.

Even though there is no callus formation and resorption, this process is not any faster than secondary bone healing. However, it is advantageous at joint surfaces or the forearm where callus formation would block movement and reduce functional outcome.

If primary bone healing fails then fixation with absolute stability will not promote callus formation. This can lead to atrophic non-union.

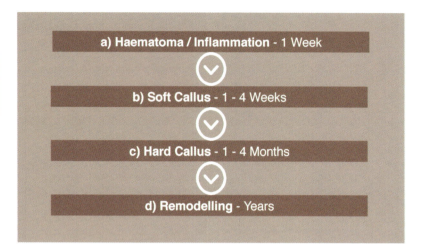

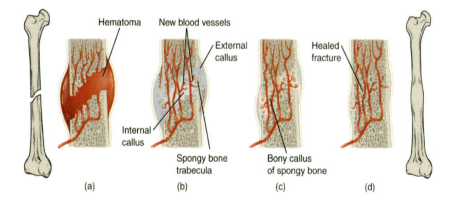

Figure 1.3 Secondary bone healing.

Secondary bone healing

If a fracture is treated without surgical input, then the natural method of fracture repair is via secondary bone healing (Figure 1.3).

Within the first week a haematoma develops. This is a fibrin clot which is replaced over time by granulation tissue. New blood vessels grow into the haematoma and osteoclasts remove any necrotic bone edges.

After the first week, the healing process becomes organised into soft callus. This is a combination of fibrous tissue, cartilage and woven bone and is visible on x-ray. After a further month, the soft callus is resorbed through a process of invasion with new blood vessels. These blood vessels bring with them osteoblast precursors, which in turn lead to hard mineralised osteoid callus.

From this point woven bone is remodelled into lamellar bone and the canal reforms.

For secondary bone healing there needs

Basic Science of Orthopaedics: Bone Healing

to be some controlled motion between the fracture surfaces under functional load. This is relative stability. This is because strain or movement at the fracture site stimulates secondary healing.

If secondary bone healing fails, a hypertrophic non-union will occur. This is the result of a good blood supply but excessive strain. This prevents progression of callus to bone and requires biomechanical stabilisation to allow callus progression to bone to occur.

Using primary and secondary bone healing

The implants used for operative fixation will provide either absolute or relative stability (Figure 1.4). Implant selection is therefore governed by the type of healing that is required.

In general:

- Primary bone healing is for intra-articular fractures or bone combinations that act like a joint (for example the forearm).

- Secondary bone healing is generally for diaphyseal fractures where the formation of callus will not impinge on movement.

A* ORTHOPAEDICS

The WHO checklist is an international form designed to prevent surgical error.

It uses 3 pauses to check, re-check and triple check the patient's identity, side of operation, planned procedure and potential complications.

In a recent systematic review a strong correlation was shown in use of checklist and reduction in mortality, complications and surgical site infection

(Bergs J, et al. Systematic review and meta-analysis of the effect of the World Health Organization surgical safety checklist on postoperative complications. Br J Surg. 2014 Feb;101(3):150–8)

Relative Stability (indirect healing)	Absolute Stability (direct healing)
• POP • IM Nail • TENS Nail • Bridging plate • Buttress plate • Ex-fix	• Lag Screw • +/- Protection Plate • Compression plate • Compression nail • TBW • Circular frame

Figure 1.4 Implants and the type of bone healing generated. Depending on how a device is used will modify the type of healing generated.

2. Pre-op planning

The pre-operative planning phase of a procedure is a vital stage in performing successful fracture fixation. It draws on the surgeon's knowledge of bone healing and the mode in which the implants will be used. It also requires an understanding of the logistics within theatre and is much more than identifying the steps from skin knife to final suture.

The preoperative plan has 3 stages: before, during and after the operative procedure and each is crucial in preventing patient harm and producing the best possible outcome for patient, surgeon and theatre staff.

Stage 1: Before procedure

Before the patient has even been sent for, the surgeon must ensure that the patient has been consented and marked appropriately. It is best practice for the surgeon to meet the patient on the ward before the list begins and this also gives an opportunity to ensure all necessary bloods have been taken and reported.

In theatre the use of a World Health Organisation (WHO) briefing is mandatory to ensure that all kit is sterile, all sizes of implants are available, the correct table in theatres and there is a plan for the administration of prophylactic antibiotics.

It is worth discussing with the anaesthetist about the planned anaesthetic and analgesia as the overall responsibility for the patient lies with the surgeon. It is worth considering what nerve blocks are indicated or contraindicated. For instance, a tibial fracture is a relative contraindication to popliteal nerve block due to the potential to mask symptoms of compartment syndrome.7

Stage 2: In theatre

When the patient is in the operating room, the most common pitfall is working out where to position the table, image intensifier and scrub team. The patient needs to be transferred safely and each hospital will have a specific policy for this. The patient needs to be positioned to give good access to the surgical field and to minimise damage to other structures. To minimise damage to soft tissues pillows / tape / padding and sandbags may be required.

It is important to ensure that the x-ray is positioned so that it can be easily seen by the operating surgeon and so two views can be obtained of the fracture and required bones. This prevents a great deal of frustration later. The fracture can then be reduced and the operation can commence.

Stage 3: After theatre

After theatre, a clear operation note should be constructed giving instructions to recovery staff and for convalescence on the ward. The operation note should include planning for: mobilisation, antibiotics, venous thromboprophylaxis, splints or frames and criteria for discharge and follow up. This facilitates a safe recovery and timely discharge.

3. Methods of fracture fixation

A wide range of implants are available to deliver absolute or relative stability to encourage fracture healing. After deciding what method of bone healing is required the next task is to select the best implant to deliver the stability required.

Plates and screws

In orthopaedics, a plate is a device designed to be held onto a bone with screws. A plate can have a wide range of roles, and the function of the plate dictates what type of stability it can deliver.

A screw is a device to convert rotational movement into linear motion. Screws come in a variety of sizes and can be fully threaded or partially threaded, self-tapping and sometimes self-drilling. In isolation, a screw can be used as a lag screw.

Lag screw

The lag screw provides a significant amount of compression to hold a fracture together and can be combined with plates to encourage primary bone healing. It is important to know the core diameter and thread diameter of the screw that you are attempting to use as a lag screw. For this example, a small fragment screw will be used with a core diameter of 2.5mm and a thread diameter of 3.5mm.

An initial gliding hole is drilled through the near cortex. This hole will have no hold and allows the screw to glide through it and is the same diameter as the threads (3.5mm). A guide is inserted into the gliding hole and the far cortex drilled to the core diameter (2.5mm) of the lag screw. Countersink, measure then tap. The depth is measured and a screw selected. The hole is tapped if required and the near cortex countersunk. On advancing the screw the fracture is compressed developing absolute stability.

Neutralisation / Protection plate

In this mode a plate is used to protect a lag screw, such as in an ankle ORIF. The plate can be lightweight as its function is to resist torsion, rather than to provide the compression to maintain anatomical reduction. In this mode it is contributing to absolute stability.

Compression Plate

For some fractures, such as in the radius or ulna, it is not possible to place a lag screw due to a transverse fracture pattern yet absolute stability is still required. In this instance a plate can be used in compression mode by careful screw placement. The fracture is reduced and held and a neutral screw drilled, measured and inserted in the centre of a hole in the plate. An eccentric hole is then drilled through the other fragment and a screw inserted. The action of the head of the screw against the edge of the hole in the plate compresses the fracture (Figure 1.5). This mode generates absolute stability.

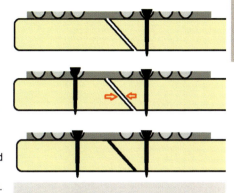

Figure 1.5 Compression of a fracture using a plate in compression mode.

Bridging plate

If a fracture is multi-fragmentary it may be advantageous to use a plate in bridging mode. Here the plate is used to span the fracture, causing minimal disruption to the blood supply in the zone of injury.

The bone needs to be restored to its original length, axis and rotation before fixation. If this is done the fracture will heal by callus formation due to relative stability from the construct.

Buttress plate

A plate can be used in buttress mode to maintain the position of a fracture to enable it to heal. The deforming forces on the fracture help reduce and compress the fragments against the plate, generating absolute stability. Examples where this mode is used include tibial plateau fractures and volar displaced distal radius fractures (Figure 1.6) where holding the fracture in place is enough to obtain reduction.

Anti-glide plate

Other less frequently used modes of plate fixation include anti-glide type of buttress plate where the plate prevents bone

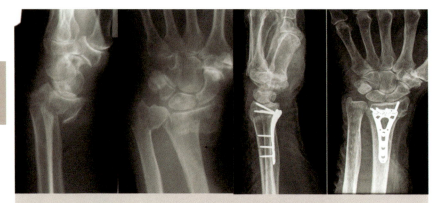

Figure 1.6 Volar displaced distal radius fracture managed with a buttress plate.

fragments from slipping out of alignment. The tension band principle will be covered later.

External fixation

External fixation can be used in several ways. An external fixator provides a rapid means of temporising a fracture to allow soft tissue regeneration before definitive fixation, or it can be a mode of definitively fixing a fracture. Crucially, it can be a method of saving a patient's life by reducing the volume for a fracture to bleed into and is therefore an essential tool in a surgeon's kit.

The indications for external fixation are:

1. Intraoperative distraction
2. Emergency stabilisation
3. Definitive fixation

In general, external fixators provide relative stability, and this stability can be altered in several ways depending on the construction of the fixator.

Intramedullary nail

The intramedullary (IM) nail is a load sharing device for diaphyseal fractures. They produce relative stability.

In order to successfully insert an IM nail careful pre-op planning is required. For femoral nails the patient has to be positioned so the surgeon can gain access to the greater trochanter. This is usually by positioning the patient with the torso in a "banana" position, with the hip adducted.

In a similar manner to bridging plates, the fracture must be reduced before the nail is passed. The bone must have its length, axis and rotation restored to produce a satisfactory outcome. There are several adjuncts available to ease reduction. An axillary crutch can be used to elevate the distal fragment and negate the action of gastrocnemius. A reduction finger can be passed through a proximally reamed shaft to guide the placement of the guide wire and an external fixator or frame can be used – as long as the pins do not interfere with the placement of the guide wire or nail.

The entry point for the nail is essential. Too medial and there is a risk of avascular necrosis to the head and too lateral and the nail will fracture the medial cortex. Nails differ in the correct entry point so it is vital to know the equipment that is being used.

Reaming increases the canal diameter but also destroys the endosteal blood supply. This is compensated for by an increase in the periosteal blood supply and reaming encourages bone growth. However bone necrosis may increase infection rate and marrow emboli are dangerous, especially following chest trauma.

As nails have become more advanced and stronger the indications for their use are expanding. They can also be used for proximal and distal metaphyseal fractures where additional locking screws or bolts are required alongside blocking (poller) screws to obtain fracture reduction The indications are likely to expand further as the technology develops.

Tension band wires

The calcium hydroxyapatite content of bone makes it very strong in axial compression. When a bone is loaded the natural curve results in a tension and compression side. The tension band works by shifting the centre of rotation to convert a tension surface into a compression surface.

In order to apply this principle, there must be full contact between the two cortical surfaces on the compression side of the bone (the side opposite to the implant). If there is communution on the compression side the implant will fail as the bending stress will cause increased implant fatigue (Figures 1.7).

Tension bands can be static or dynamic. A dynamic tension band increases the compressive forces on the fracture when the joint is moved, such as in a patella or olecranon repair. A static configuration exerts continuous compression, such as in a medical malleolus fixation.

Further reading

1. AO E-learning. www.aofoundation.org

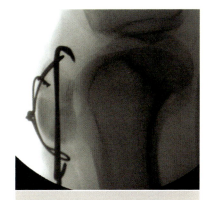

Figure 1.7a Tension band wiring of a patella: post-op radiograph

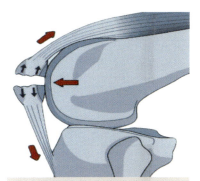

Figure 1.7b Tension band wiring of a patella: distracting muscle forces

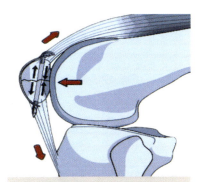

Figure 1.7c Tension band wiring of a patella: TBW compressive forces

Chapter 2

Chapter 2: The Trauma Call

Managing Severe Trauma and Orthopaedic Emergencies

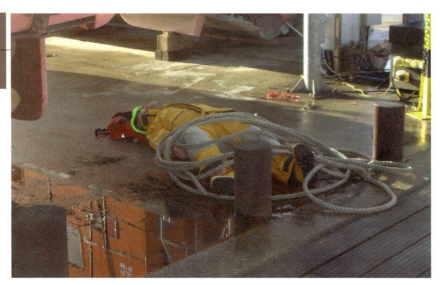

Chapter 2: The Trauma Call Contents

1. Trauma call: an introduction — p25
2. Preparation — p25
3. Primary survey — p26
4. Secondary survey — p27
5. Damage control — p30

3 Topics Not To Miss

1. Compartment syndrome
2. Hidden injuries
3. Occult blood loss

Trauma Checklist

Handover from pre-hospital	• Identify team and make introductions • Discuss skills of each team member • Assign roles • Mechanism of injury • Identify likely injuries • Theatre, radiology, blood bank
Primary Survey (A)	• Is airway patent? • Can the airway be managed with a bag valve mask or does the patient need a more definitive airway? • C-spine immobilised? • Any catastrophic haemorrhage requiring tourniquet?
Primary Survey (B)	• Trachea position • Oxygen saturations • Air entry • Percussion note
Primary Survey (C)	• Blood pressure and heart rate • IV access and send bloods (FBC, U&Es, lactate, clotting, glucose, crossmatch) • Heart sounds • Consider giving blood products if in hypovolaemic shock. May need massive transfusion protocol
Primary Survey (D)	• Pupils • AVU or GCS
Primary Survey (E)	• Log roll • Abdominal exam • Long bones • Consider pelvic binder if mechanism suggestive of fracture

Trauma Checklist Continued

Secondary Survey Head	• Blood on scalp • CSF from nose or ears • Racoon eyes or battles sign • Deviated nose or septal haematoma
Secondary Survey Spine	• Pain on palpation • Range of movement • Low threshold for CT and keep immobilised
Secondary Survey Limbs	• Deformity • Normal movements • Pain on palpation
Secondary Survey Trunk	• Injuries or bruising front or back • Urine dip for haematuria • Rib fractures or flail chest
Secondary Survey Neuro	• Upper and lower limb power, tone, sensation and reflexes • PR exam

Always Remember:

1. Open fractures
2. Compartment syndrome
3. Beware of hidden injuries in an unconscious patient

Within 10 minutes the team should have decided:

1. Straight to theatre?
2. Straight to CT scan?
3. Safe for observation?

1. Trauma call: an introduction

Trauma calls require different skills to those traditionally taught in medical school. These patients are often very unwell, and need a co-ordinated effort from a slick multi-disciplinary team to prevent death or major complications. There is not time to produce a full clerking, and the important steps are to first identify life and then any limb threatening issues that need to be managed now.

Your first trauma call

With the development of the UK trauma network, most district general hospitals are managing severe trauma much less frequently than before. However, it is still possible for major trauma to be stabilised and packaged in a smaller hospital's emergency department before transfer to a larger centre.

Advanced Trauma Life Support (ATLS) is an international course designed by the America College of Surgeons and helps trainees prepare for trauma situations, usually where they are the only doctor available to lead a small team. Its European counterpart, the European Trauma Course is more focussed on the integrated team. Both are great courses to do while in the early years of training where the system and sequence provides a solid foundation on which to base your practice.

As an easy to remember guide, trauma calls can be divided into 3 phases. The first is preparation, where it is vital to establish a solid team. The second is the primary survey, investigations and decision. This is the lifesaving part of the sequence. Finally comes the secondary survey, management and rehabilitation.

2. Preparation

In this phase of the trauma call, you have an opportunity to demonstrate non-technical skills as the team forms. Expect to see representation from the following departments:

- Emergency department (usually team leader)
- General surgery
- Trauma and orthopaedics
- Anaesthetics, an operating department practitioner
- Nursing staff, including a timekeeper and scribe.

While there are some characters that are vital to a trauma team, there are also members who have different levels of experience and confidence. In one hospital that I have worked in, the surgical team was represented by the on-call houseman. This "surgeon" was only months out of medical school and had a very different skill set to other teams where the surgical input is from a registrar or consultant.

Top tips include writing your name on the apron in large letters to improve communication, and liaise with theatres and radiology so you know what resources are available. It is vital to assign a leader and everyone needs to know who is in charge.

Your preparation phase gives the team time to digest the pre-alert and to formulate a plan of attack and assign roles. Be prepared to be adaptable to the situation in front of you, and work hard on communicating all findings clearly and concisely to the team via the team leader.

Chapter 2

3. Primary survey, investigations and decision

In trauma, the primary survey is the screening tool for identifying life threatening injuries. This information allows you to decide if the patient needs to have a CT scan, or go straight to theatre to control bleeding.

Airway, catastrophic bleeding and c-spine

The framework in the assessment checklist should be familiar to most trainees, with some tweaks on the standard ATLS protocol. Airway, cervical spine protection and evaluation of catastrophic bleeding are the priority steps as airway or profuse bleeding will kill your patient and c-spine transaction will result in long-term disability. Management does not need to be massively invasive as the airway can be managed with simple manoeuvres such as the jaw thrust and getting a good seal with a bag-valve mask (this may take two hands, especially if the patient is sporting a beard).

It is useful to learn how to perform a surgical airway as a back-up measure. Catastrophic bleeding may be controlled with direct pressure or by the application of a tourniquet. If a tourniquet is applied, write the time the tourniquet was applied on the tourniquet and on the limb to ensure the tourniquet is not left on for too long.

Breathing and circulation

Breathing and circulation assessments are tailored to identify and manage pneumothorax, haemothorax and tamponade. At this stage check that you have seen a full set of observations and that a set of bloods have been sent including a crossmatch for 4 units, FBC, U&E, coagulation and lactate. Examine the patient looking for sources of bleeding – a tender abdomen, dull chest or angulated limbs. Do not spring the pelvis; it does more harm than good as you can dislodge the clot that is preventing the patient from exsanguinating. Instead, if you suspect a pelvic fracture then apply a binder and request x-rays or CT. Look at the observations; is there evidence of hypovolaemic shock?

Any trauma patient with evidence of shock should be assumed to be hypovolemic until proved otherwise. There is some debate between the UK and ATLS guidelines as to how to proceed. ATLS guidelines currently recommend giving up to 2L of crystalloid or colloid before reaching for blood. Conversely, experience from recent military conflicts suggests that patients fare better when blood and blood products (platelets and fresh frozen plasma) are infused early. The use of these blood products will be included in your hospital's massive transfusion policy; it is worth finding and reading this in case you have to activate it.

Disability, exposure and decision

A baseline assessment of disability can be achieved with a quick Glasgow Coma Score (often on the trauma documentation) and checking the pupils. Check the limbs for obvious wounds and if you do not suspect a pelvic fracture then arrange for a log roll to evaluate the spine, inspect the back and perform a digital rectal examination.

Once you have gathered all of this information and are ready to decide what to do, the next 3 options tend to be available. 1) The patient is unstable and needs to go to theatre for laparotomy or external fixator, 2) the patient is relatively stable and needs a CT to identify injuries 3) the patient is completely stable and the team can proceed to a secondary survey. The major trauma centre target to arrive at this decision is 10minutes from the time the patient arrived in the Emergency Department.

4. Secondary Survey

The secondary survey is the opportunity to identify any injuries that may have been missed in the primary assessment. It is the part of the trauma call most often delegated to the orthopaedics team, and requires a thorough assessment when the patient is not distracted by other injuries. It may immediately follow the primary assessment, or follow lifesaving treatment. Some patients, if intoxicated when injured, will even need to wait for the morning to sober up.

The secondary survey is summarised within the assessment checklist and requires evaluation of every bone that might be injured and requesting imaging as required.

Orthopaedic Injuries

Major trauma can result in virtually any injury. However, the emergencies that will require you to get the boss to see the patient are listed below.

Compartment syndrome

This is an orthopaedic emergency. Compartment syndrome is a process where the pressure within a myofascial compartment exceeds the perfusion pressure of that compartment. This can be caused by factors external to the compartment, such as a tight cast or skin contractures following a burn, or by internal factors such as swelling following a fracture or blunt injury.

The presenting feature is pain, pain and more pain. The pain will be out of proportion to the injury sustained. Review the drug card to see how much pain relief has been given – it is usually lots. The pain is usually within the muscle compartment rather than at the fracture site and is exacerbated on passive stretch of the muscle. Other features are late and herald that the compartment syndrome has been missed. A lack of pulses suggests a vascular injury and need to be documented and an opinion

Airway, catastrophic bleeding and c-spine

Breathing
Haemo/Pneumothorax?

Circulation
Hypovolaemic shock
Bloods
Observation

Disability
AVPU
Pupils

Exposure
Abdominal exam
Long bones
Spine

Decision
Theatre
CT scan
Observe + secondary survey

Chapter 2

from a vascular surgeon obtained. A pale palor and paraesthesia indicate tissue ischaemia and the need to get a good lawyer.

If you suspect compartment syndrome, take a quick history and make the patient nil by mouth in anticipation of surgery. Cut any cast, dressing or splint down to skin – do not leave any wool or padding as this alone can cause significant pressure. Keep the limb at the level of the heart, high elevation will reduce the perfusion pressure while dangling the limb low will increase swelling. Give a dose of morphine and call the registrar. If the pain does not resolve with these conservative measures then the patient will need to go to theatre for a fasciotomy.

It is useful to know how to measure compartment pressures, which can be found in the skill station. Compartment pressures are useful when the patient is unconscious following major injury or cannot give a pain response. Compartment syndrome is present if the pressure is more than 30mmHg, or the Δp (diastolic blood pressure – compartment pressure) is less than 30mmHg.

INITIAL MANAGEMENT FOR SUSPECTED COMPARTMENT SYNDROME:

- Complete assessment checklist
- Split plaster down to skin
- Give dose of opiate pain killers
- Recheck after 10 minutes
- Consider compartment pressures if patient unconscious
- Prepare patient for theatre for fasciotomy

ADMISSION REQUIRED IF:

Always. Bed rest with limb at level of heart

ORTHOPAEDIC EMERGENCY:

Time to wake up the registrar ASAP

Open fractures

Increasingly, open fractures are being managed on daytime trauma lists, rather than as emergency cases overnight. An open fracture is any fracture that communicates with the skin, and includes in-out fractures where the bones have protruded and returned to their original position and graphic injuries that look dreadful.

The British Orthopaedic Association and British Association of Plastic, Reconstructive and Aesthetic Surgeons have released joint guidelines of managing open fractures in the lower leg which can be applied to most open fractures anywhere in the body. These standards may be found online, and are included in the initial management box.

INITIAL MANAGEMENT FOR OPEN FRACTURE:

- Complete assessment checklist:
- i. Give broad spectrum antibiotics (co-amoxiclav, cefuroxime or clindamycin IV) within 3h of injury
- ii. Assess Neurovascular status regularly, especially after any manipulation
- iii. Rush to emergency theatre if evidence of vascular injury or compartment syndrome or if wound contaminated by marine, agricultural or sewerage material
- iv. Pre-operative planning should be completed by plastics and orthopaedics
- v. In the Emergency Department
- a. Remove gross contamination
- b. Photograph wound
- c. Dress with saline soaked swabs
- d. Splint the limb to include the knee and ankle (for tibial fractures)
- Consider transfer to tertiary referral unit where combined orthopaedics and plastics input is available

Trauma Call: Secondary Survey

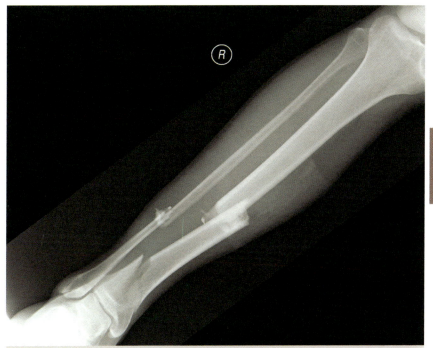

Figure 2.1 Open fracture of tibia and fibula following motorcycle crash. Note dressing over wound to mid-shin. This is a high energy injury with a high risk of compartment syndrome, despite the open wound.

ORTHOPAEDIC EMERGENCY:

Time to wake up the registrar:

1. Evidence of vascular injury.
2. Marine, agricultural or sewerage contamination
3. Unstable fracture requiring reduction that cannot be achieved in ED

ADMISSION REQUIRED IF:

Always. May need transfer to unit with plastic surgeons for combined management

Chapter 2

5. Damage control orthopaedics and early total care

If the patient needs to go to theatre tor fracture management, the injuries can be managed with damage control or early total care. Damage control is as it sounds: performing lifesaving surgery to splint and minimise further harm to the patient. The plan is to provide definitive fixation after a period of rest. This allows the soft tissues to settle and for the trauma response and physiology to return to normal. This reduces the chance of developing a systematic inflammatory response and death.

In contrast, early total care means that all fractures are fixed, wounds covered and the patient allowed to start their rehabilitation much sooner. Many consultants will have tales of operating through the night on such patients in epic procedures. This is less common now, as in order to safely perform early total care the following criteria need to be met. These criteria are shown below.

These criteria should also be measured during the operation. It is possible that during a long operation one or more of these may become abnormal requiring a change from early total care to damage control.

Further reading

1. Carlino W. Damage control resuscitation from major haemorrhage in polytrauma. Eur. J. Orthop. Surg. Traumatol. 2014; 24 :137–41.

2. Schäfer N, Driessen A, Fröhlich M, Stürmer EK, Maegele M, TACTIC partners. Diversity in clinical management and protocols for the treatment of major bleeding trauma patients across European level I Trauma Centres. Scand. J. Trauma. Resusc. Emerg. Med. 2015; 23 :74.

3. Ali AM, McMaster JM, Noyes D, Brent AJ, Cogswell LK. Experience of managing open fractures of the lower limb at a major trauma centre. Ann. R. Coll. Surg. Engl. 2015; 97 :287–90.

Trauma Call: Damage Control Orthopaedics

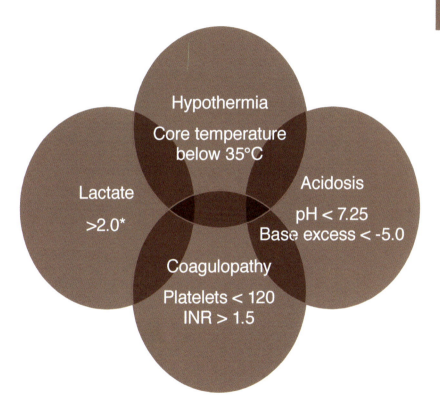

Figure 2.2 Contraindications for performing early total care in a multiple injured patient.
*If early total care is to be considered, lactate may be greater than 2.0 but should be trending downwards.

Chapter 2

TRAUMA CALL

SKILL STATION: MEASUREMENTS OF COMPARTMENT PRESSURES (LOWER LEG)

Indication:	• Suspicion of compartment syndrome in an obtunded patient
Team Required:	• 1 person to administer block
Preparation:	• Acquire compartment pressures transducer or set up and zero an arterial line transducer
Equipment:	• Skin marker. Chlorhexidine skin prep. Pressure transducer

STEP 1: Identify sites for measurement

Mark planned puncture sites and prep skin with chlorhexidine. Suggested puncture sites are:
1. anterior compartment – 1cm lateral to the anterior border of tibia
2. lateral compartment – 0.5cm anterior to the posterior border of fibula
3. superficial posterior – most posterior point of the calf
4. deep posterior – 0.5cm posterior to the medial border of the tibia

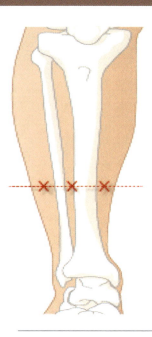

32

STEP 2: Insert needle

Insert the needle perpendicular to the skin at the marked sites to the following depths to reach the compartment.

1. Anterior compartment –3cm
2. Lateral compartment –1cm
3. Superficial posterior –3cm
4. Deep posterior –2-4cm towards the fibula

(Red lines are needles)

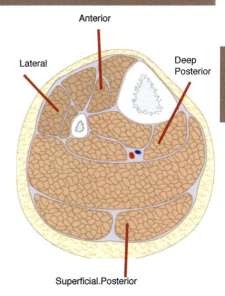

STEP 3: Measure pressures

Compartment syndrome is diagnosed if the absolute pressure of any of the four compartments is greater than 30mmHg or if the relative pressure is within 30mmHg of the patient's diastolic blood pressure

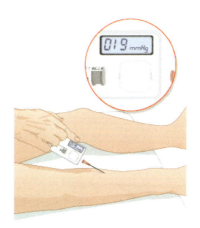

Chapter 3

Chapter 3: Upper Limb

Shoulder, Humerus, Elbow, Forearm and Distal Radius

Chapter 2: Upper Limb Contents

1. Distal radius fracture	p38	4. Humerus fracture	p42
2. Forearm fracture	p40	5. Dislocated shoulder	p44
3. Elbow fracture	p41	6. Other Presentations	p46

UPPER LIMB

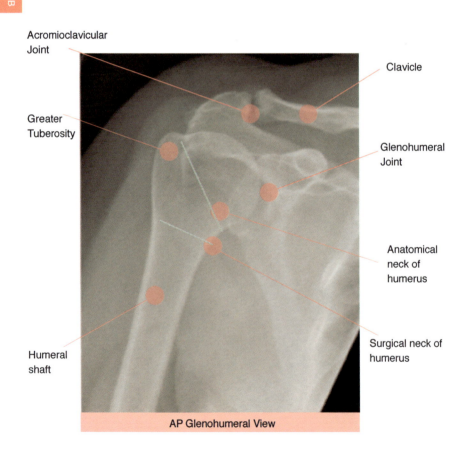

- Acromioclavicular Joint
- Clavicle
- Greater Tuberosity
- Glenohumeral Joint
- Anatomical neck of humerus
- Surgical neck of humerus
- Humeral shaft

AP Glenohumeral View

34

Upper Limb

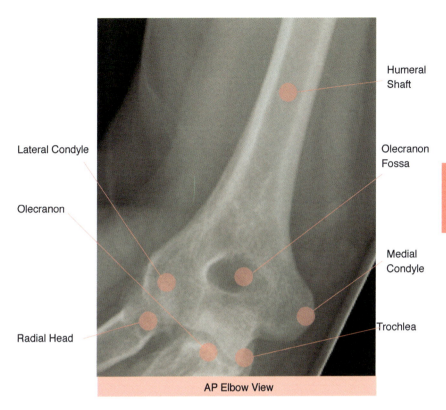

AP Elbow View

3 Topics Not To Miss

1. Humeral shaft fracture with wrist drop
2. Posterior dislocated shoulder
3. Don't forget to examine the neck

Injuries to the upper limb are common as individuals try and use the limb to break their fall and protect the rest of their body. With advancing age, osteoporotic fractures become increasingly likely and provide a substantial workload for the emergency department. Fortunately, many of these injuries do not require emergency admission, and can be managed on a semi-elective basis via fracture clinic.

Chapter 3

Upper Limb Assessment Checklist (History)

Injury (Site)	• Left or Right • Wrist • Forearm • Elbow • Upper arm • Shoulder / clavicle • Other
Mechanism Associated injuries	• Open • Closed • Other injuries
Past Medical History	• Handedness (Left or Right) • Past Medical History • Drugs and allergies • Last meal • Occupation

Upper Limb Assessment Checklist (Examination)

Observation	- Deformity - Wounds
Neurological Power	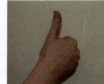 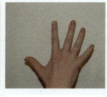 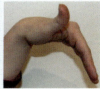 Radial nerve Ulna nerve Median nerve
Neurological Power	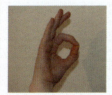 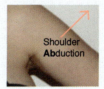 Anterior interosseous Axillary nerve
Hand Sensation (And Document Pulses)	- Radial - Ulna - Median - Check pulses 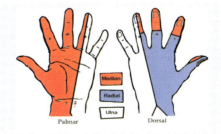

Chapter 3

1. Distal radius fracture (adult)

Fractures to the distal radius are incredibly common, with an incidence of 36.8 per 10,000 person years in women over 35 in the UK. The most common mechanism is a fall on an outstretched hand (FOOSH), such as in placing a hand on the ground to break a fall. There are two peaks in the presentation of these fractures: in the young due to high energy injuries and in the elderly due to osteopenia. Treatment varies markedly between these two groups.

Fractures to the distal radius are divided into volar displaced and dorsal displaced depending on the direction of the displacement to the distal fragment. Volar displaced fractures may be referred to as Smiths type if the fracture is extra-articular or as a Volar Bartons if the fracture is intra-articular. These fractures are inherently unstable due to the strong pull of the flexor tendons, and require operative fixation with locking or buttress plate.

A* ORTHOPAEDICS

The Lafontaine criteria can be applied to dorsally displaced (Colles type) fractures to determine if the fracture is unstable. These are:

1. Dorsal angulation > 20°
2. Dorsal comminution
3. Initial displacement > 1cm
4. Initial radial shortening > 5mm
5. Associated ulna fracture
6. Severe osteoporosis

The more unstable, the more likely operative management is required. These criteria can also be applied to check if a reduction is adequate.

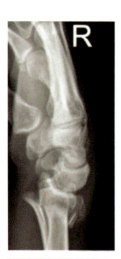
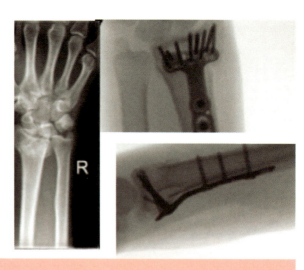

Figure 3.1a-d Dorsal displaced intra-articular fracture, treated with a distal radius volar locking plate

Upper Limb: Distal Radius Fracture

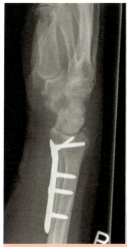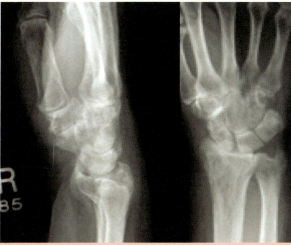

Figure 3.2a-c Volar displaced intra-articular fracture, treated with a distal radius volar locking plate

Dorsally displaced fractures give the textbook "dinner fork" deformity that was described by Colles in 1814 These fractures are more stable than the volar displaced fractures and may be managed conservatively. However, it the fracture is unstable then it may need operative management. Generally, this will take the form of manipulation under anaesthesia and k-wire fixation if the fracture is extra-articular and can be reduced with a closed manipulation. Otherwise, a plate fixation (ORIF) is necessary. It is wise to council the patient and consent for both as this is not always decided until theatre.

INITIAL MANAGEMENT FOR CLOSED DISTAL RADIUS FRACTURE:

- Complete assessment checklist
- Manipulation in Emergency Department with Bier's block or Haematoma block
- Application of plaster (below elbow backslab for dorsally displaced, above elbow volar slab for volar displaced)
- Check x-ray
- Recheck neurovascular status
- Home if safe with fracture clinic follow up

ORTHOPAEDIC EMERGENCY: TIME TO WAKE UP THE REGISTRAR

Neurovascular compromise – the fracture fragments may cause a secondary carpal tunnel syndrome which requires careful observation and elevation

ADMISSION REQUIRED IF:

- Unable to cope at home (may require admission under geriatric / general medical team)
- Open injury (see trauma call chapter)

Chapter 3

2. Forearm fractures

In orthopaedics, the forearm is regarded as a joint. This is because the interaction of the radius and ulna at the proximal and distal radio-ulna joints permits pronation and supination movements, and explains why many of these fractures require operative fixation.

As well as acting as a joint, the forearm is a ring – rather like a Polo mint. The two bones are connected by strong ligaments at wrist and elbow. If you try and break it, it will fail in two places. This makes it near impossible to get a displaced, isolated fracture of only one of the bones. It is possible to get an isolated comminuted fracture of the ulna from a high-energy direct blow. These are known as nightstick fractures and are named after the police truncheons that may, in cases of over-enthusiasm, have lead to this injury.

More commonly the forearm ring breaks in two places. This could be a fracture of both radius and ulna, or a failure of proximal or distal radial-ulna joints. These have eponymous names, and invariably need fixing.

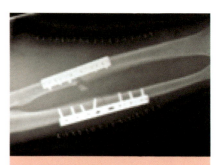

Figure 3.4 Midshaft radius and ulnar fractures treated with ORIF

A* ORTHOPAEDICS

Eponymous fractures to the forearm are favourites in the morning trauma round. They are best remembered by recalling football teams that play in blue and red:

Manchester United: Monteggia fracture: Ulna fractures (radial head dislocates)

Glasgow Rangers: Galeazzi fracture: Radius fractures (ulna dislocates at distal radial-ulna joint).

INITIAL MANAGEMENT FOR CLOSED FOREARM FRACTURE:

- Complete assessment checklist – don't forget to examine the elbow and wrist
- Application of above elbow plaster backslab
- Check x-ray
- Recheck neurovascular status
- Admit for elevation and observation

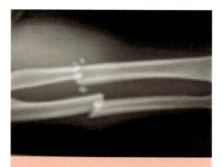

Figure 3.3 Midshaft radius and ulnar fractures treated with ORIF

Upper Limb

ADMISSION REQUIRED IF:

- Routine

ORTHOPAEDIC EMERGENCY: TIME TO WAKE UP THE REGISTRAR

- Neurovascular compromise
- Compartment syndrome – expect lots of swelling. (See orthopaedic emergencies chapter)

3. Elbow fractures

At the elbow, 3 bones articulate to provide movement. These are the radial head, olecranon (ulna) and distal humerus. Each of these can be broken during a fall.

Radial head fractures

These may be sustained during a fall on an outstretched hand as the force is transmitted from the hand to wrist to elbow. The radial head impacts against the capitellum and fractures. Accordingly, the classification for these fractures is grade 1: undisplaced fracture, 2: two part fracture as a chunk of the radial head sheers off during the injury and 3: comminuted fracture as the radial head explodes on impact. Un-displaced fractures are often managed conservatively, where-as displaced or comminuted fractures will be fixed with open reduction internal fixation or excised and replaced with a prosthesis.

These fractures do not usually warrant admission unless there is an elbow dislocation which requires investigation.

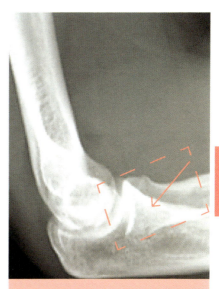

Figure 3.5 Lateral x-ray of elbow with an un-displaced radial head fracture (arrow). Note the anterior and posterior fat pad where the fat has been displaced (making it visible) by the haemarthrosis.

A* ORTHOPAEDICS

The radial head helps to stabilise the elbow, especially against valgus force. The "Terrible Triad" (very unstable elbow) is:

1. Radial head fracture
2. Coronoid fracture
3. Elbow dislocation (often with lateral collateral ligament injury)

These injuries have poor outcomes and require operative stabilisation.

Chapter 3

Olecranon fractures

Olecranon fractures are sustained by falling directly onto the elbow. The fracture pattern may be a simple two part fracture, or a configuration with multiple fragments and comminution. The initial management of these fractures is straightforward and follows a similar pattern to other upper limb injuries. Definitive treatment for these fractures is usually surgical but may be conservative dependent on age, fracture pattern and patient co-morbidities and functional status. As the fracture is intra-articular absolute stability is required which can be achieved with a tension band or plate fixation.

INITIAL MANAGEMENT FOR CLOSED OLECRANON FRACTURE:

- Complete assessment checklist
- Analgesia
- Above elbow plaster backslab if required for analgesia – may be comfortable in broad arm sling
- Recheck neurovascular status
- May be discharged home to wait for an operation or may be admitted

ADMISSION REQUIRED IF:

- Unable to cope at home
- Pre-operative assessment or space on theatre list (depending on local protocol)

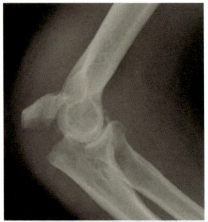
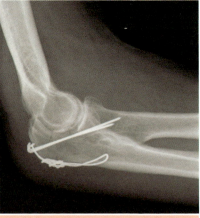

Figure 3.6 a, b Olecranon fracture treated by tension band wire

Distal humeral fractures (adult)

In adults, distal humeral fractures are usually intracondylar and occur most frequently in young men and older women. These fractures are intra-articular and without anatomical reduction and fixation are likely to result in substantial loss of joint movement.

Management of these fractures in the elderly is controversial, with the decision between operative management involving open reduction internal fixation or a total elbow replacement. Conservative management, the "bag of bones" strategy, relies on the soft tissues holding the bones roughly approximated allowing healing in whatever position they rest in. Although historical, it may still be used in patients unift for surgery.

INITIAL MANAGEMENT FOR CLOSED DISTAL HUMERUS FRACTURE:

- Complete assessment checklist
- Analgesia
- Collar and cuff or above elbow backslab for comfort
- Recheck neurovascular status
- May be discharged home to wait for an operation or may be admitted

ADMISSION REQUIRED IF:

- Unable to cope at home
- Pre-operative assessment or space on theatre list (depending on local protocol)

4. Humerus fractures

Humeral fractures can be to the proximal humerus, humeral shaft or distal humerus. Distal humeral fractures are discussed in the elbow fractures section. Both proximal humeral and humeral shaft fractures are unlikely to require admission from the Emergency Room, and most can be managed conservatively.

Proximal humeral fractures

Fractures to the proximal humerus may be associated with dislocations to the humeral head. With this in mind scrutinise the x-rays carefully and ensure that you have two orthogonal views to review. There are many options for the radiographer to obtain a decent lateral image of the gleno-humeral joint. If you are unsure from the original x-rays then give the patient analgesia and discuss with the radiographers alternative x-ray positions to obtain better images. Initial management of proximal humeral fractures is with a collar and cuff to use gravity to pull the elbow down and align the proximal humerus. They can then be reviewed in fracture clinic where many will continue conservative management. Operative management is for selected patients only, mainly young patients or for isolated indications such as displaced greater tuberosity avulsions. A large recent randomised controlled trial (PRoFHER) showed a limited role for surgery in the elderly patient.

INITIAL MANAGEMENT FOR CLOSED PROXIMAL HUMERUS FRACTURE:

- Complete assessment checklist
- Analgesia
- Collar and cuff
- Recheck neurovascular status
- Fracture clinic follow up

ADMISSION REQUIRED IF:

- Unable to cope at home (may require admission under geriatric / general medical team)

Chapter 3

Humeral shaft fractures

Humeral shaft fractures are often dramatic on x-ray. Twisting injuries will cause spiral fractures to the humerus which may or may not have an accompanying butterfly fragment.

Of particular concern with these fractures is the radial nerve. This structure is closely applied to the humerus as it winds down in the spiral groove and may be injured or stretched when the bone breaks.

Fortunately, most of these fractures heal with conservative management. Initial management involves using gravity to pull the arm down and the fracture back into alignment. This can be achieved with a collar and cuff or plaster slab.

INITIAL MANAGEMENT FOR CLOSED HUMERAL SHAFT FRACTURE:

- Complete assessment checklist
- Analgesia
- Collar and cuff, humeral brace or hanging U plaster slab
- Recheck neurovascular status
- Check x-ray
- Fracture clinic follow up

ADMISSION REQUIRED IF:

- Unable to cope at home (may require admission under geriatric / general medical team)

ORTHOPAEDIC EMERGENCY: TIME TO WAKE UP THE REGISTRAR

- Neurovascular compromise – look for a wrist drop

5. Dislocated shoulder

Shoulder dislocations are a common presentation following shoulder injury. In order to permit the wide range of motion that the shoulder enjoys the glenoid has to be shallow which makes this joint prone to dislocation. As a rule of thumb, the earlier in life you sustain your first dislocation the more likely it is to dislocate again. An anterior dislocation is more common than a posterior dislocation.

The typical presentation is of a patient with asymmetrical shoulders who is unable to move the dislocated arm. A good screening test is to ask the patient to touch his good shoulder with the hand on the painful arm. If he is able to do this then a dislocation is unlikely.

Remember to get two views of the shoulder as a posterior dislocation is not always apparent on the anterio-posterior views. A posterior dislocation is an unusual injury. Patients may dislocate posteriorly during a fit and this may be missed for several days unless you have a high index of suspicion.

Do not forget to assess the neurovascular status prior to any reduction manoeuvre – pay particular attention to the axillary nerve (sensation over regimental badge area and abduction of the shoulder) and musculoskeletal nerve (elbow flexion and sensation to lateral forearm.

Upper Limb: Dislocated Shoulder

INITIAL MANAGEMENT FOR CLOSED DISLOCATED SHOULDER:

- Complete assessment checklist
- Analgesia
- Reduce shoulder ASAP – this will require sedation from Emergency Department or anaesthetics
- Recheck neurovascular status
- Check x-ray. If it remains dislocated consider re-manipulation or admission
- Fracture clinic follow up

ADMISSION REQUIRED IF:

- Unable to reduce: admit for closed +/- open reduction in theatre

ORTHOPAEDIC EMERGENCY: TIME TO WAKE UP THE REGISTRAR

- Cannot relocate shoulder in ED

A* ORTHOPAEDICS

There are many techniques for reduction of anterior dislocated shoulders. This requires some form of analgesia and / or sedation. Two favourites are:

1. Kochers: i. Abduct the arm to 60°

ii. Externally rotate to 90°

iii. Adduct arm across chest

iv. Internally rotate arm

2. Modified Hippocratic:
Inline traction: one person applying in-line traction to dislocated arm, one providing counter traction with a folded sheet around the axilla.

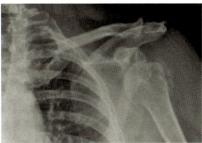
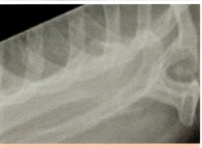

Figure 3.7 a, b AP and axillary view of anterior dislocated shoulder, with glenoid fracture and fracture to the greater tuberosity. This fracture could not be reduced closed, and needed reduction and stabilisation in theatre.

Chapter 3

Initial treatments of other common presentations

- **Clavicle fracture**

    Symptoms and signs: Pain over clavicle following landing on arm. Unable to abduct shoulder.

    Investigation: X-ray (one view usually sufficient)

    SHO management: Broad arm sling. Check for skin tenting.

    Definitive management: Needs fixing if very displaced or skin tenting. Some choose to fix clavicles to get patients back to normal function sooner, especially if the patient needs to do a lot of work overhead.

- **Frozen shoulder (adhesive capsulitis)**

    Symptoms and signs: Unable to move shoulder. No fracture on x-ray. Normal bloods.

    Investigation: x-ray to exclude fracture and bloods to help exclude infection

    SHO management: Analgesia and reassure

    Definitive management: Usually conservative. Some will see a shoulder specialist and have a manipulation under anaesthesia or surgical release of the capsule.

- **Biceps tendon rupture (distal)**

    Symptoms and signs: Often patients with large muscles. Feels a 'pop' and has reduced power in supinating forearm

    Investigation: Diagnosis is usually clinical.

    SHO management: Analgesia in the Emergency Department and refer to upper limb fracture clinic

    Definitive management: May be reattached surgically

- **Biceps tendon rupture (proximal)**

    Symptoms and signs: Traumatic rupture gives the "Popeye" deformity of the upper arm

    Investigation: Diagnosis is usually clinical

    SHO management: Analgesia in the Emergency Department and refer to upper limb fracture clinic

    Definitive management: Usually conservative

- **Greater tuberosity fracture**

    Symptoms and signs: Pain in shoulder following fall, may have associated dislocation

    Investigation: x-ray

    SHO management: Collar and cuff for comfort. Will need discussion with a shoulder surgeon and fracture clinic follow up

    Definitive management: Requires surgical fixation of displacement > 5mm due to the pull of supraspinatous

- **Olecranon bursitis**

    Symptoms and signs: Bulging inflammatory sac around olecranon

    Investigation: X-ray to exclude osteomyelitis and bloods to help rule out infection and septic arthritis

    SHO management: Confirm no infection by examination and investigation. If infected admit for antibiotics, if not can be discharged with analgesia and sling

Definitive management: Usually conservative

Gout and pseudogout

Symptoms and signs: Can present in any joint and mimic septic arthritis

Investigation: Serum urate (may be normal in an acute flare), inflammatory markers will be mildly raised. Crystals on joint aspirate are diagnostic
SHO management: Initial investigations and joint aspiration

Definitive management: 3-4 days of non-steroidal anti-inflammatory drugs or colchicine. Repeat flares may need treatment with allopurinol (usually started by rheumatology or GP).

Further reading

1. Rangan A, Handoll H, Brealey S, Jefferson L, Keding A, Martin BC, et al. Surgical vs Non-surgical Treatment of Adults With Displaced Fractures of the Proximal Humerus. JAMA. 2015;313(10):1037.

2. Costa ML, Achten J, Parsons NR, Rangan A, Griffin D, Tubeuf S, et al. Percutaneous fixation with Kirschner wires versus volar locking plate fixation in adults with dorsally displaced fracture of distal radius: randomised controlled trial. BMJ. 2014;349:g4807.

3. Lafontaine M, Hardy D, Delince P. Stability assessment of distal radius fractures. Injury. 1989;20(4):208–10.

Chapter 3

UPPER LIMB

SKILL STATION: REDUCTION OF DISTAL RADIUS FRACTURE WITH HAEMATOMA BLOCK

Indication:	• New dorsal displaced distal radius fracture.
Team Required:	• 1 person to reduce and mould • 1 person to apply counter tracton • 1 person to apply plaster
Preparation:	• Gain consent • Draw up 10ml local anaesthetic (e.g. 10ml 1% lidocaine) • Prep dorsum of wrist with chlorhexidine or bethadine
Equipment:	• Plaster trolley • Luke-warm water

STEP 1: Advance needle into haematoma

Advance needle into haematoma, located by palpating fracture. Confirm position by aspirating haematoma before injecting. Wait 10 minutes for local to take effect

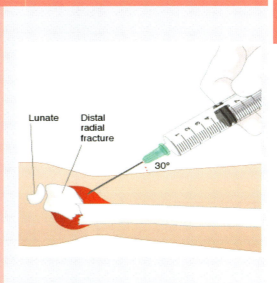

Chapter 3

UPPER LIMB

STEP 2: Apply wool and prepare plaster

Position by having assistant hold distal humerus. Elbow should be flexed to 90 degrees. Confirm that the person designated to apply plaster is ready and ask them to apply a single layer of wool.

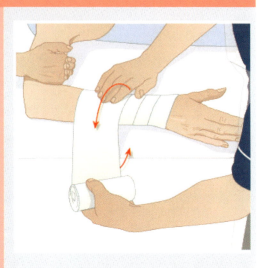

STEP 3: Reduce fracture

Hold thumb, index and middle fingers and apply in-line traction to reduce the fracture. Keep your arms straight and lean back while your assistant provides counter traction.

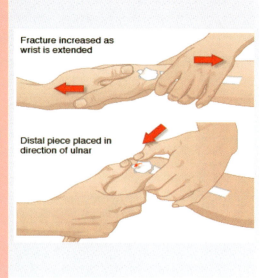

Upper Limb

STEP 4: Dis-impact the fracture

It may be necessary to dis-impact the fracture. This is done by extending the wrist at the fracture site, applying additional traction and returning the hand to a flexed, ulna deviated position.

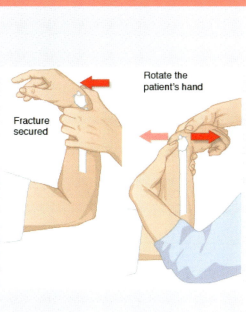

Fracture secured

Rotate the patient's hand

STEP 5: Apply moulded plaster

Hold the position while plaster is applied. Mould the plaster by squeezing above and below the fracture to ensure good, firm contact with the skin.

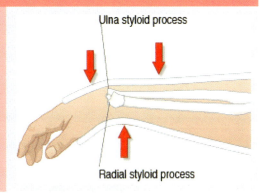

Ulna styloid process

Radial styloid process

Chapter 4

Chapter 4: Hands

Metacarpal, Phalangeal and Carpal Bone Injuries

Chapter 4: Hands Contents

1. Metacarpal fractures	p55	4. Tendon injuries	p60
2. Carpal bone fractures including dislocations around the lunate	p58	5. Flexor sheath infection	p61
		6. Other Presentations	p62
3. Nail bed injury	p60		

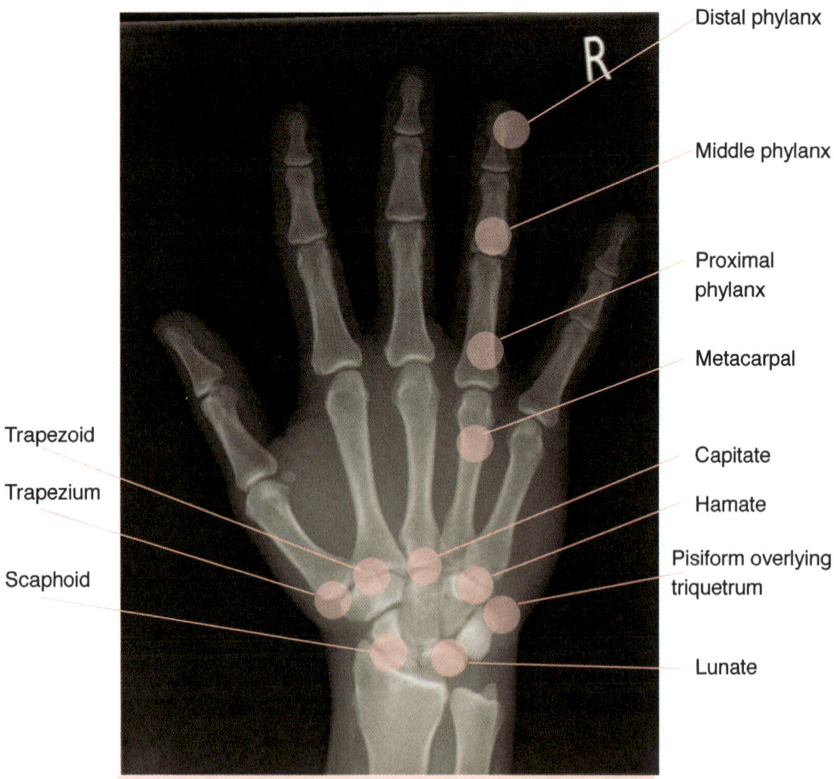

HANDS

- Distal phylanx
- Middle phylanx
- Proximal phylanx
- Metacarpal
- Capitate
- Hamate
- Pisiform overlying triquetrum
- Lunate
- Trapezoid
- Trapezium
- Scaphoid

AP Hand View

Hand Assessment Checklist (History)	
Presenting Feature (History)	• Age • Time of injury
Mechanism	• How injury sustained • Likelihood of infection
Patient factors	• Left or right handed • Occupation
Past medical history	• Diagnoses • Medications • Allergies
Examination: Look	• Compare right to left • Swelling • Deformity
Examination: Feel	• Specific areas of tenderness • Swelling over joints
Examination: Move	• Test all joints and tendons

Chapter 4

Hand Assessment Checklist (Tendon Examination)

Flexor digitorum profundus (FDP)	• Function: Flexes finger at DIPJ
Flexor digitorum superficialis (FDS)	• Function: Flexes finger at PIPJ
Flexor pollicis longus (FPL)	• Function: Flexes thumb at IPJ
Extensor digitorum (ED)	• Function: Extends fingers
Flexor pollicis brevis (FPB)	• Function: Flexes thumb at CMCJ
Abductor pollicis brevis and longus (AbPL / AbPB)	• Function: Abducts thumb

Rotational stability assessment (Clinical not radiological)

Assess cadence/ cascade and flexion	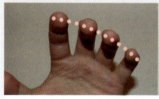 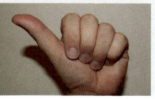 Normal Cadence Normal flexion

Hand Assessment Checklist (Neurovascular Examination)

Neurological Power

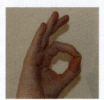
Median nerve (AIN)

Radial nerve

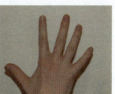
Ulna nerve

Neurovascular Sensation & Pulses
- Radial
- Ulna
- Median

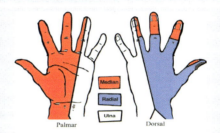

3 Topics Not To Miss

1. Dislocations – always get a lateral x-ray
2. Fight bites
3. Digital nerve injuries in innocent looking wounds

1. Metacarpal fractures including fracture dislocations and fight bites

Metacarpal Fractures

Metacarpal fractures are exceptionally common. Injuries to these bones present regularly to the Emergency Department. Invariably they occur in young men who have either fallen over onto a fist, or alternatively hit someone or something…

In the hand, the metacarpals of the index and middle fingers are attached to the rest of the hand and wrist by strong, stiff ligaments. In contrast, the metacarpals for the ring and little finger are much more mobile. This makes the ring and index finger metacarpals more prone to fracture. The metacarpal can fracture at the neck – a boxer's fracture, in the shaft or at the base. A shaft fracture is often a spiral fracture and may be unstable. Fractures to the base are intra-articular and may be associated with dislocation.

Chapter 4

For all of these fractures, an assessment of rotational stability needs to be undertaken, as this will dictate management. Look at the cadence of the fingers compared to the other hand, and the direction at which the finger points when it is flexed. A rotationally unstable finger will produce a dramatic deformity, and often requires operative management. Initial management for a closed metacarpal fracture (without dislocation) is dependent on patient pain. Often, a simple buddy strap will suffice to splint the fractured finger so that healing can occur. If a cast is required then it should be in the Edinburgh position. This is a slab applied to the volar surface of the forearm that extends to the proximal interphalangeal joints. The wrist is extended and the metacarpophalangeal joints are flexed at 90°.

This reduces the tension on the intrinsic muscles and prevents the fingers from becoming stiff. Patients with these fractures should be re-examined in fracture clinic (ideally a hand clinic) to confirm stability. If they are unstable then they will be listed for fixation with screws and plate or k-wires.

INITIAL MANAGEMENT FOR METACARPAL FRACTURES (CLOSED WITH NO DISLOCATION)

- Complete assessment checklist
- Analgesia
- Assess rotational stability
- Obtain PA, oblique and lateral x-ray
- Buddy strap or volar plaster slab in Edinburgh position

ADMISSION REQUIRED IF:

- Rotational instability

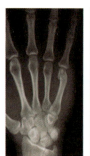
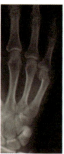
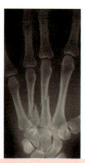
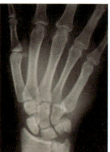
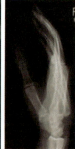

Figure 4.1 Left to right: 1) PA and oblique fracture showing neck of 5th metacarpal fracture. 2) Spiral fracture of 3rd and 4th metacarpal 3) Fracture and dislocation of 4th and 5th metacarpals – note the indistinct joint line on the PA view.

Carpometacarpal Dislocations

Dislocation of the ring and little finger carpometacarpal joints may occur when significant axial load is placed on a flexed ring and little finger. The x-ray appearance is of an indistinct joint on the PA film, and the dislocation is seen most clearly on the lateral view.

In this fracture dislocation, the fracture may run through the base of the metacarpals, or be an avulsion fragment from the hamate. As with all dislocations an attempt should be made to reduce the dislocation in the Emergency Department with appropriate analgesia and sedation. However, these injuries are very unstable and it is likely that the dislocation will re-occur despite an adequate reduction (often before the patient gets to the check x-ray). These injuries need admission for stabilisation. This is usually achieved with k-wire fixation.

INITIAL MANAGEMENT FOR CLOSED CARPOMETACARPAL JOINT DISLOCATION

- Complete assessment checklist
- Analgesia
- Obtain PA, oblique and lateral x-ray
- Reduce dislocation with analgesia and sedation
- Dorsal plaster back slab
- Check x-ray

ADMISSION REQUIRED IF:

- Most need admission for k-wire stabilisation

Fight Bites

Fight bites are the result of a patient's hand colliding with another person's mouth. The human mouth is rich in bacterial flora and so 10-15% of wounds that have been contaminated by the mouth will become infected.

The wound is usually overlying the knuckle on the dorsum of the hand, and may extend to the tendon or through the joint capsule.

These injuries are serious as they invariably lead to unpleasant infections. The patient will need admission for antibiotics and possibly washout of the infected tissue and joint.

A fight bite in conjunction with a metacarpal fracture is a serious open fracture and antibiotic selection will need to be discussed with the local microbiology team. These will require admission for stabilisation of the fracture and washout of all infected tissue.

From experience, many patients will present to the emergency department and not admit to having punched another person. However, if they are questioned directly and understand the implications of a human bite infection then they often give a more detailed history.

INITIAL MANAGEMENT FOR FIGHT BITE WITH OR WITHOUT UNDERLYING FRACTURE

- Complete assessment checklist
- Analgesia
- 3. Obtain PA, oblique and lateral x-ray
- IV antibiotics as per local policy
- Check tetanus status and administer anti-tetanus immunoglobins if indicated
- Volar plaster slab in Edinburgh position

ADMISSION REQUIRED IF:

- Requires IV antibiotic therapy
- Fracture identified

2. Carpal bone fractures including lunate and peri-lunate dislocations

Scaphoid Fracture

The most important of the carpal bone fractures to be aware of are fractures to the scaphoid. Injury to the scaphoid occurs during a fall onto an outstretched hand and may accompany a fracture to the distal radius. Scaphoid fractures present with tenderness in the anatomical snuff box and should be imaged by obtaining scaphoid views.

If a fracture is identified then the patient should be immobilised in a scaphoid cast. Distal fractures are usually managed non-operatively whereas proximal pole fractures have a high non-union rate and high risk of avascular necrosis. Waist fractures are more controversial, and may be managed operatively or non-operatively.

Importantly, if no fracture is seen on the scaphoid views then the patient should be splinted and reviewed in 10-14 days with repeat x-rays as the fracture line may not become visible until this follow up film.

Other fractures to bones in the carpus are uncommon and can be managed in the first instance with a backslab and be followed up in hand or fracture clinic.

INITIAL MANAGEMENT FOR SUSPECTED SCAPHOID FRACTURE

- Complete assessment checklist
- Analgesia
- Obtain scaphoid view x-ray
- If fracture identified then treat in scaphoid cast and review in (hand) fracture clinic
- If no fracture identified the treat in futura splint and re-xray in clinic in 10-14 days

ADMISSION REQUIRED IF:

- Not required acutely

Perilunate Dislocation

When reviewing patients with injuries to the wrist it is worth being aware of the normal articulations between the wrist and carpus. Normally the wrist is made up of a capitate articulating within the moon shaped lunate which in turn articulates in the lunate fossa of the distal radius.

A perilunate dislocation occurs when the capitate is displaced out of the lunate, and represents a substantial soft tissue injury. This is a very unstable injury and should be manipulated into the best possible position in the emergency department and then admitted for ligament reconstruction and joint stabilisation on the first available list.

Lunate Dislocation

A lunate dislocation may occur with the lunate being forced in a volar or dorsal direction. Again, this represents a significant soft tissue injury and there may be an associated fracture of the lunate or scaphoid. An attempt may be made to reduce this in the Emergency Department but this injury will require admission for open reduction, fixation and ligament reconstruction.

Hands: Carpal Bone Fractures

Figure 4.2 Lunate and Perilunate dislocations

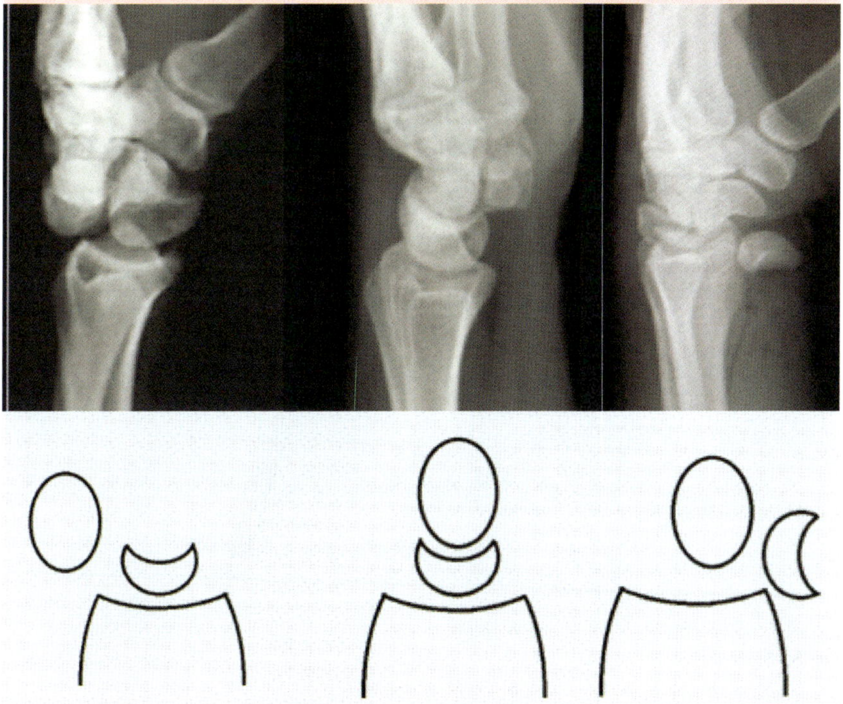

Peri-lunate dislocation | Normal wrist | Lunate dislocation

INITIAL MANAGEMENT FOR PERILUNATE OR LUNATE DISLOCATION

- Complete assessment checklist
- Analgesia
- PA and lateral x-ray
- Attempt reduction with analgesia
- Dorsal plaster back slab
- Recheck neurovascular status
- Check x-ray

ADMISSION REQUIRED IF:

- All cases

ORTHOPAEDIC EMERGENCY: TIME TO WAKE UP THE REGISTRAR

- Evidence of neurovascular compromise or carpal tunnel syndrome

3. Nail bed injury

An intact nail bed is required to allow the nail to grow smoothly. However, it is often injured by dropping heavy items onto the hand or by shutting the finger in a door, or even by running miniature tractors over the digit. As the distal phylanx is closely associated with the nail bed, it is also often fractured if the nail bed is disrupted, leading to an open fracture.

These patients need a ring block and washout in ED to reduce the risk of infection. For many of them, a nail bed repair can be completed at the same sitting removing the need for an admission and a trip to theatre. Further details as to how to repair the nail bed is included in this chapter's skill station.

If the injury is too severe to be managed in the ED, or if the patient will not cope with the procedure outside of theatre (such as in most paediatric cases) then admit the patient with broad spectrum IV antibiotic cover and prepare them for theatre.

INITIAL MANAGEMENT FOR NAIL BED INJURIES

- Complete assessment checklist
- Analgesia and ring block
- Washout and nail bed repair
- Finger dressing
- Discharge home with oral antibiotics

ADMISSION REQUIRED IF:

- Unable to tolerate nailbed repair in ED

4. Tendon injuries

Injuries to the flexor or extensor tendons are identified by evaluating the function of each tendon as part of your examination. When there is a wound it is possible to explore in the emergency department with local anaesthetic. If you do so, beware – the tendon may have been injured while the digit was in flexion or extension and the laceration will move to a position which is not necessarily under the wound when the finger is moved. A tendon injury over a joint with an overlying wound is likely to indicate joint involvement, so have a low threshold of admitting these patients for washout in theatre.

INITIAL MANAGEMENT FOREXTENSOR OR FLEXOR TENDON INJURY

- Complete assessment checklist
- Analgesia
- IV antibiotics
- Check tetanus status and administer anti-tetanus immunoglobins if indicated
- Immobilise with a dorsal slab for volar injuries or a volar slab for dorsal injuries

ADMISSION REQUIRED IF:

- Routine for antibiotics, elevation and early repair

5. Flexor tendon infections

The flexor tendons in the hand require good tensile strength and a smooth tunnel to glide through to generate optimal function and grip strength. Infection within the flexor sheath of the fingers can rapidly lead to damage of the normally smooth apparatus of the pulleys and sheaths and cause fibrosis of the tendon sheaths and thus cause rapid and irreversible loss of function.

It is worth remembering that the flexor sheath of the little finger communicates with the ulna bursa and the sheath of the thumb communicates with the radial bursa. It is possible for infections in these digits to track into the palm of the hand and form a horseshoe abscess as two bursae join at the carpal tunnel. The most common cause is inoculation from a direct overlying wound, and there may be a delay to presentation as the infection develops.

Flexor tendon infection may result in reduced function from scar tissue or from tendon rupture. Initial management is therefore geared towards preparing the patient for theatre for washout.

ADMISSION REQUIRED IF:

- All cases

ORTHOPAEDIC EMERGENCY: TIME TO WAKE UP THE REGISTRAR

- Call to confirm if patient needs to go to theatre overnight

A* ORTHOPAEDICS

Diagnosis of flexor tendon infection may be aided by looking for the 4 Kanaval's signs.

These are:

1. Finger held in flexion
2. Pain on passive extension
3. Fusiform (sausage-like) swelling of the finger
4. Pain on palpation of the flexor tendon.

INITIAL MANAGEMENT FOR FLEXOR TENDON INFECTION

- Complete assessment checklist
- Analgesia
- Bloods and blood cultures
- Elevate in Bradford or similar sling
- Consider antibiotics if patient septic – try and hold off until cultures obtained in theatre

Chapter 4

Initial treatments of other presentations

- **Dupyten's contracture**

Symptoms and signs: Fixed flexion of MCPJ or PIPJ with palpable band in hand

Investigation: Diagnosis is clinical

SHO management: Refer to hand clinic if patient symptomatic

Definitive management: Conservative, injection or surgical release

- **Trigger finger**

Symptoms and signs: Finger catches on flexion and has to be straightened by other hand

Investigation: Diagnosis is clinical

SHO management: Refer to hand clinic if patient symptomatic

Definitive management: Conservative or surgical release

- **Carpal tunnel syndrome**

Symptoms and signs: Numbness in distribution of median nerve, worse at night or when driving. Positive tinnels or Phalens test (symptoms reproduced when wrist extended for 30s or carpal tunnel percussed for 15s)

Investigation: Diagnosis is often clinical, may require nerve conduction studies to prove source of symptoms

SHO management: Refer to hand clinic if patient symptomatic

Definitive management: Conservative, injection or surgical release – will need urgent surgical decompression if due to trauma

- **Phalangeal fractures**

Symptoms and signs: Pain, swelling and deformity

Investigation: x-ray PA, lateral and oblique. Check not open injury.

SHO management: Buddy strap and refer to hand fracture clinic. If mallet finger (unable to extend DIPJ due to tendon avulsion) then use a mallet splint to rest the tendon and instruct the patient not to take it off at all.

Definitive management: Conservative for many, surgical for unstable fractures or subluxed fragments.

- **Amputations**

Symptoms and signs: partial amputation or fingers in a bag

Investigation: x-ray hand. Wrap amputated fingers in damp gauze and place in a bag of ice

SHO management: Complete amputation: discuss with plastics or hand team for possible re-implantation, otherwise admit for debridement and terminalisation if not salvageable

Definitive management: Some may be treated conservatively but many need surgical debridement

Further reading

Hart RG, Kleinert HE. Fingertip and nail bed injuries. Emerg. Med. Clin. North Am. 1993; 11 :755–65.

Neuhaus V, Jupiter JB. Current concepts review: carpal injuries - fractures, ligaments, dislocations. Acta Chir. Orthop. Traumatol. Cech. 2011; 78 :395–403.

SKILL STATION: NAILBED REPAIR

INDICATION	• Crush injury to distal finger with nail bed injury
TEAM REQUIRED	• 1 person to repair nail bed • 1 person to assist (if available)
PREPARATION	• Gain consent – ensure the patient is aware of risk of infection and of pits or ridges to the nail
EQUIPMENT	• Obtain: suture kit with needle holder, scissors and blunt clip (e.g. artery clip). 4.0 nylon and 6.0 vicryl. 2L saline • Draw up 10ml local anaesthetic (e.g. 10ml 1% lidocaine. Do not use local with adrenaline) • Prep web space (for ring block) with chlorhexidine or bethadine

Chapter 4

HANDS

STEP 1: Digital ring block

Perform a digital ring block by infiltrating approximately 4ml local anaesthetic to the ulna and radial side of the finger, at the level of the netacarpophalanegal joint. Also inject over the top of the joint to block the dorsal nerve. Wait 10 minutes for the local to take effect.

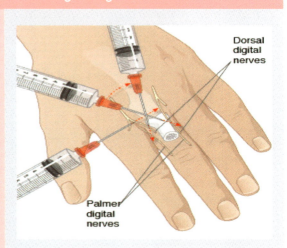

STEP 2: Apply tourniquet and remove nail

Apply a finger tourniquet (one can be made by cutting a finger off a small glove). Elevate the nail by sliding the blunt clip under the nail and spreading. Be careful not to cause any additional injury to the nail bed. You may need to grasp the edges of the nail and roll them out to release the nail from the skin folds. Remove the nail and store in a sterile pot of saline

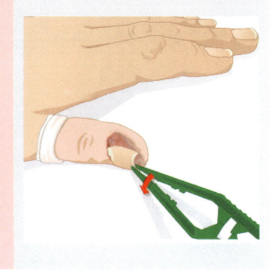

Hands: Nailbed Repair

STEP 3: Wash nail bed

Wash the nail bed with the sterile saline. You may want to do this over a sink to minimise mess. Repair the nail bed with interrupted 6.0 dissolvable sutures

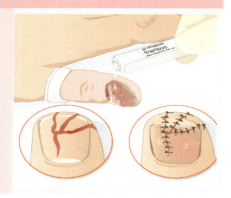

STEP 4: Repair nail edges

Repair the skin edges with interrupted 4.0 non-absorbable sutures. Trim any frayed edges from the nail that was removed and reimplant under the nail fold to keep it open. Hold in place with a figure of 8 non-absorbable suture over the top.

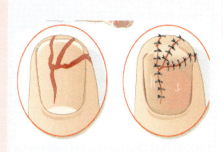

STEP 5: Remove tourniquet and apply dressing

Remove the tourniquet and apply a finger dressing. These often ooze so use a non-stick dressing underneath some gauze and bandage. The patient may be discharged with a course of oral antibiotics and a fracture clinic review in 10 days to check the wound and remove the sutures. Warn the patient that the nail will fall off- but a new one should grow in its place.

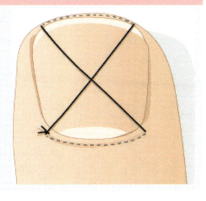

Chapter 5

Chapter 5: Lower Limb

Femur, Knee, Tibia and Ankle Injuries

Chapter 5: Lower Limb Contents

1. Femoral fractures	p69	4. Tibial shaft fractures	p76
2. Knee injuries	p70	5. Ankle fractures	p77
3. Tibial plateau fractures	p75	6. Other Presentations	p79

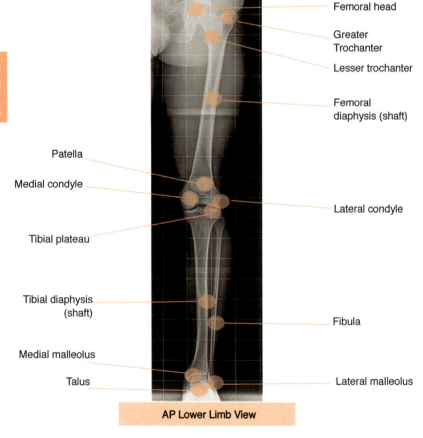

AP Lower Limb View

Lower Limb Injury Assessment Checklist (History and Examination)

Injury Site (History)	• Left or Right • Foot • Ankle • Knee • Thigh • Hip • Other
Injury (History)	• Mechanism
Associated injuries	• Open • Closed • Other injuries
Past Medical History	• Past Medical History • Drugs and allergies • Last meal • Occupation
Examination Observation	• Deformity • Wounds
Lower Limb Power	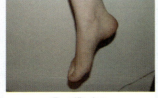 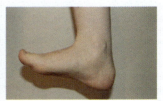 Dorsiflexion Plantarflexion

Chapter 5

Lower Limb Injury Assessment Checklist (Senation and Vascular)

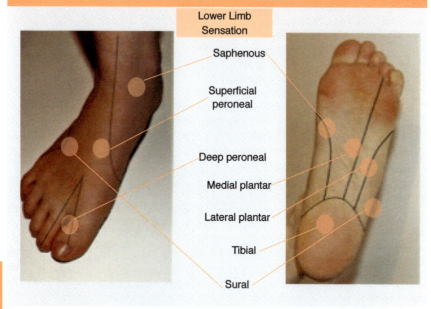

Lower Limb Sensation
- Saphenous
- Superficial peroneal
- Deep peroneal
- Medial plantar
- Lateral plantar
- Tibial
- Sural

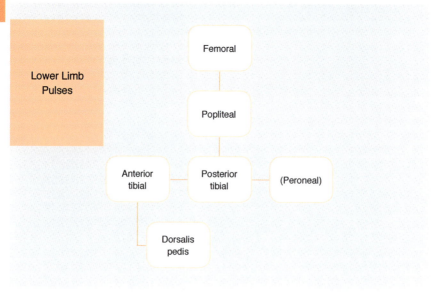

Lower Limb Pulses
- Femoral
- Popliteal
- Anterior tibial
- Posterior tibial
- (Peroneal)
- Dorsalis pedis

3 Topics Not To Miss

1. Dislocated knee with popliteal artery damage
2. Displaced ankle fracture
3. Polytrauma or spine injury

1. Femoral fractures

Femoral fractures can be proximal, shaft or distal. Proximal femoral fractures, around the neck of femur, are discussed in detail in the hip fracture chapter. Shaft fractures are generally high energy injuries, whereas distal femoral fractures may be high or low energy.

Femoral shaft fractures

Fractures to the diaphysis (shaft) of the femur are serious injuries, regardless of the mechanism. They are often associated with other injuries, so the patient should be assessed in a systematic manner like in the trauma call chapter. Once life threatening injuries have been identified and managed, a simple measure to prevent further blood loss is the application of a Thomas splint.

There are several splints available, each with advantages and disadvantages. It is worth finding out the local preference in your hospital and also how to apply a standard Thomas splint as shown in the skill section in the paediatric chapter. This standard method, while old fashioned, allows for traction to be applied for 24-48 hours and can be converted to balanced traction of a definitive operation needs to wait for kit or a particular surgeon.

Diaphyseal fractures can cause significant internal bleeding. Splinting will help this but you will also need to monitor the patient's parameters and resuscitate with fluids or blood products as necessary.

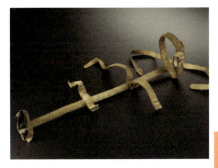

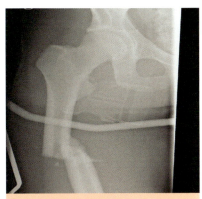

Figure 5.1 a, b Thomas leg splint as used between 1901-1920 (still in use today!) and transverse femoral fracture, treated initially in a modern metal Thomas splint.

In general, diaphyseal fractures are fixed with intramedullary nails. However, if the fracture is particularly distal then fixation with a plate may be selected in preference. Either way, the mode of fixation is with relative stability. The advantage of using a nail is that the patient can mobilise and weight bear straight away.

INITIAL MANAGEMENT FOR CLOSED FEMORAL FRACTURE

- Complete assessment checklist
- Consider femoral nerve block
- Application of Thomas splint
- Check x-ray
- Recheck neurovascular status
- Bloods including FBC, U&E and Group and save

ADMISSION REQUIRED IF:

- Pre-op

ORTHOPAEDIC EMERGENCY: TIME TO WAKE UP THE REGISTRAR

- Neurovascular compromise
- Open injury or part of polytrauma

Distal femoral fractures

Distal femoral fractures may be intraarticular or extra articular. Intraarticular fractures have a fracture that extends between the condyles, though this may be difficult to identify on the original X-rays.

In the emergency department it is often tempting to put these fractures into an above knee backslab. This is often done poorly, if the top of the cast finishes at the fracture site all it will achieve is hinging the fracture and causing additional displacement. A wiser idea is to apply skin traction and admit the patient.

An above knee plaster can always be applied tomorrow by the orthopaedic technicians in the plaster room.

The initial evaluation of these fractures requires careful assessment of patient factors, with documentation of mobility, demand and past medical history. In the elderly, it may be a better option to perform a primary distal femoral replacement, with the associated risks of further fracture and need for revision. Alternatively the fracture can be fixed with a plate or if it is an extraarticular fracture with a retrograde nail.

INITIAL MANAGEMENT FOR DISTAL FEMORAL FRACTURE

- Complete assessment checklist
- Analgesia
- Application of skin traction or above knee backslab
- Check x-ray
- Recheck neurovascular status
- Bloods including FBC, U&E and Group and save
- Consider CT scan to confirm if intraarticular

ADMISSION REQUIRED IF:

- Pre-op

2. Knee injuries

Injuries around the knee that do not involve the tibial plateau or distal femur may well be a soft tissue injury or a patella fracture. These can be deceptive – it is possible to dislocate a knee during an injury and then have it reduce pre-hospital. This leads to massive ligament damage and can be associated with neurovascular injury (sometimes even limb threatening) or compartment syndrome. These knee injuries will be managed as below.

Soft tissue knee

Soft tissue knee injuries represent a spectrum from simple sprains that can be managed conservatively to major ligament injury that requires reconstruction. These are often seen in the Emergency Department, placed in a brace (Richards' or Cricket Pad) and sent home with crutches to be seen in the acute knee clinic.

Twisting injuries to the knee can produce a variety of injuries. Initial clinical examination is often limited to determining if there is an effusion or not (indicative of intraarticular pathology). Immediate swelling is suggestive of ACL rupture, whereas a meniscal injury is more likely if the onset of effusion is delayed. Further examination is usually impossible due to pain. However, when the pain and swelling has improved the following structures can be tested. The initial management of these injuries is to identify potential ligament injuries, splint and organise follow up with the knee clinic. A MRI may be useful in demonstrating the injury and to allow for early surgery if possible. The exception to this is if there is evidence of a knee dislocation.

Knee Structures and Clinical Tests

Structure	Clinical Tests
Anterior Cruciate (ACL)	• Lachmanns • Pivot shift
Posterior Cruciate (PCL)	• Posterior sag • Posterior draw
Medial Collateral (MCL)	• Opening of the joint with valgus stress with 10-20° flexion
Lateral Collateral (MCL)	• Opening of the joint with varus stress with 10-20° flexion
Posterior Collateral (PCL)	• Dial test - >10°external rotation at 10 and 90° flexion indicates PCL and posterolateral corner injury

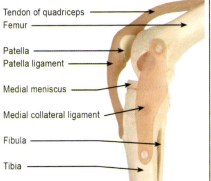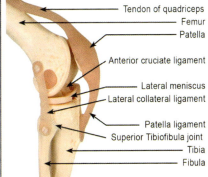

Figure 5.2 Structures around the knee

Knee dislocation

A dislocated knee is a high energy event and suggests substantial injury to the soft tissues. The tibia tends to translate anteriorly, and this puts significant stretch on the popliteal artery and common peroneal nerve. It is also possible to produce a small intimal tear in the popliteal artery which goes on to develop a full dissection. Neurovascular compromise is therefore not uncommon and needs to be identified on initial examination and reviewed regularly. A CT arteriogram of the popliteal artery is useful in identifying any damage to this vessel.

A dislocated knee should be reduced in casualty and placed in an above knee backslab. The swelling will be significant so the patient should be admitted for observation and investigation to identify soft tissue injuries that may need reconstruction. Pulses should be felt throughout the admission and observed carefully. A low threshold should be maintained for calling the vascular surgeons if there is evidence of any damage to the popliteal artery.

ORTHOPAEDIC EMERGENCY: TIME TO WAKE UP THE REGISTRAR

- Dislocation that cannot be reduced in ED
- Pulseless foot or any evidence of neurovascular compromise

INITIAL MANAGEMENT FOR SOFT TISSUE KNEE INJURY (NO DISLOCATION)

- Complete assessment checklist
- Evaluate ligaments as possible
- Apply extension splint (Richard's or Cricket Pad splint)
- Mobilise non-weight bearing
- Follow up in acute knee or fracture clinic
- Home if safe with crutches

ADMISSION REQUIRED IF:

- Unable to cope at home
- Avulsion injury to tibial spine

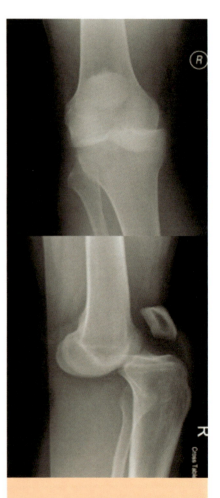

Figure 5.3 AP and Lateral radiographs demonstrating anterior right knee dislocation

Lower Limb: Knee Injuries

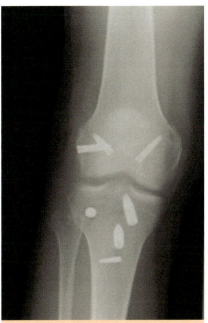

Figure 5.4 Radiograph following reconstruction of ACL, PCL + PLC

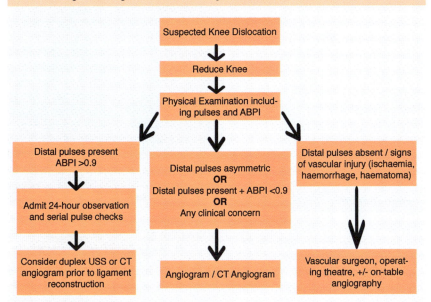

Figure 5.5 Algorithm for the management of acute knee dislocations

Chapter 5

Patella fractures

Patella fractures occur due to a direct blow to the knee. This may be caused by landing on the knee or by an impact. A longitudinal fracture may be stable and still allow the patient to straight leg raise. This indicates the extensor mechanism is intact and the patient may be treated conservatively. Equally, a transverse fracture with minimal displacement may also have sufficient strength in the retinaculum that the extensor mechanism is functional and conservative management possible. However, if the patient is unable to straight leg raise, it indicates that the extensor mechanism has failed and is now acting purely to distract and displace the fracture. These need to be fixed surgically.

Fixation options are with open reduction and internal fixation. Tension band wiring is usually successful for two part fractures, and may need reinforcing with a cerclage wire if the fracture is commented. Fixation can also be achieved with special plates for the patella.

INITIAL MANAGEMENT FOR PATELLA FRACTURE

- Complete assessment checklist
- Document neurovascular status
- Analgesia
- Apply cylinder cast
- Check x-ray

ADMISSION REQUIRED IF:

- If patient unable to straight leg raise
- Fracture displaced requiring fixation

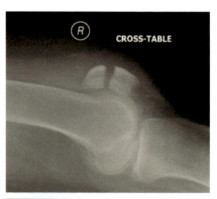
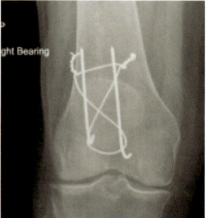
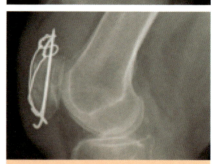

Figure 5.6 Patella fracture managed with tension band wire

Lower Limb: Tibial Plateau Fractures

3. Tibial plateau fractures

Plateau fractures are caused when the femur impacts into the tibia with force, such as in a fall onto the knee or in a road traffic collision. They are often innocent looking injuries on the first X-ray, and look much more significant on the CT and represent a significant step in the articular cartilage.

There is often a soft tissue and ligament injury associated with these fractures which needs evaluation ideally pre and post fixation.

Low energy fractures are seen in the elderly and may be fragility fractures like distal radial fractures and hip fractures. If they are undisplaced and involve only the lateral plateau they may be managed conservatively. More displaced fractures may be managed with fixation. Primary joint replacement is reserved for elderly patients with severe fractures, but gives good outcomes in smashed plateaus.

Severe fractures in the young represent high energy injuries. Bear in mind that these injuries are soft tissue events with a coincidental broken bone. This means that the knee will swell and swell and swell. It is possible for the swelling to become so substantial that the patient develops compartment syndrome or surgical fixation becomes near impossible. In this case a quick spanning external fixation may prove invaluable to reduce swelling and promote soft tissue recovery.

INITIAL MANAGEMENT FOR TIBIAL PLATEAU FRACTURES

- Complete assessment checklist
- Document neurovascular status
- Analgesia
- Apply extension splint or above knee backslab
- Consider CT

ADMISSION REQUIRED IF:

- Routine for observation

ORTHOPAEDIC EMERGENCY: TIME TO WAKE UP THE REGISTRAR

- Compartment syndrome
- Evidence of neurovascular compromise

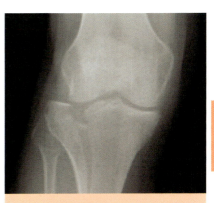

Figure 5.7 Tibial plateau fracture

A* ORTHOPAEDICS

The Schatzker classification is used to describe tibial plateau fractures. This classification ranges from 1-6 based on fracture pattern:

1. Lateral plateau split
2. Lateral plateau split and depression
3. Lateral plateau depression
4. Medial plateau fracture
5. Lateral and medial plateau fracture
6. Plateau fracture with fracture line extending to diaphysis

Chapter 5

4. Tibial shaft fractures

Tibial shaft fractures are frequently exciting injuries in that they tend to have sporting mechanisms and long stories attached! Try not to fall into the emergency department trap of getting an X-ray of an obviously broken leg before reduction. These X-rays will have an AP view of the knee captured with a lateral view of the ankle. If you think that the leg is obviously broken, and the foot and knee are facing different directions then give some analgesia and correct the alignment before the first x-ray. Not only does this make you look slightly foolish if you fail to do so when presenting at the trauma meeting, but it also reduces the time to restore normal perfusion to the foot. Failure to do so will cause a degree of neurovascular impairment.

Initial management will include documentation of neurovascular status, as well as an evaluation of other injuries and conformation as to if this is an open or closed injures. Open tibial fractures need antibiotics and management as described into the trauma call chapter. Tibial shaft fractures need reduction with plenty of analgesia and placing into an above knee backslab. For most, admission will be necessary for elevation and observation overnight to ensure compartment syndrome does not develop. The mainstay of surgical management of these fractures is with tibial nails. Some may be managed conservatively in a plaster if the fracture is not displaced. Alternatively, very distal fractures may need plate fixation if there is not space to place the distal locking bolts.

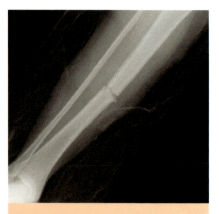

Figure 5.8 Transverse tibial shaft fracture

INITIAL MANAGEMENT FOR CLOSED TIBIAL SHAFT FRACTURE

- Complete assessment checklist
- Analgesia
- Apply above knee backslab with a social reduction – make sure the foot is pointing the same way as the knee
- Recheck neurovascular status
- Check x-ray
- Admit

ADMISSION REQUIRED IF:

- For elevation and observation

ORTHOPAEDIC EMERGENCY: TIME TO WAKE UP THE REGISTRAR

- Evidence of compartment syndrome
- Neurovascular injury

4. Ankle fractures

Ankle fractures are common, with inversion and eversion injuries occurring in the young falling on a Friday night and the old tripping while looking for the loo in the early hours.

On arrival in the emergency department, many ankle fractures will be reduced as they are obviously deformed before x-ray. If the x-ray demonstrates the ankle is subluxed or dislocated, then reduction needs to be performed as soon as possible to prevent soft tissue compromise. This is performed using the technique described in this chapter's skill section. For ankle fractures you need to establish if they are stable or unstable. A stable fracture will not displace, i.e. the talus will not slip out of joint when weight is applied to it and can be managed conservatively. Conversely, an unstable fracture will cause rapid ankle arthritis if the talus is displaced by even a few millimetres.

Different classifications are available to help you decide if an ankle is stable or not. The Lauge-Hansen classification and the AO classification are complex and not particularly reproducible, leaving the Danis-Weber classification. This classifies fractures based on the position of the fracture to the fibula. A Weber A has a fracture distal to the syndesmosis, B is a fracture at the syndesmosis and C is above the syndesmosis. A simple modification adds the damage to the medial side with 0 (no injury or tenderness), 1 (medial malleolus fracture or deltoid ligament rupture/tenderness) and 2 (posterior malleolus fracture).

Operative fixation is usually with lag screws and a neutralisation plate for Weber B 1 or 2 fractures, though a bridging plate may be required for Weber C fractures. The posterior malleolus needs to be reduced and fixed if a substantial portion of the joint is involved. Historically, a substantial portion meant 1/3 of the articular surface, but many surgeons are now fixing these fragments even if less than 1/3 of the joint is involved.

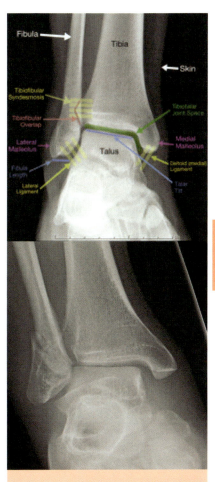

Figure 5.9 Talar shift in an subluxed ankle fracture requiring urgent reduction

Chapter 5

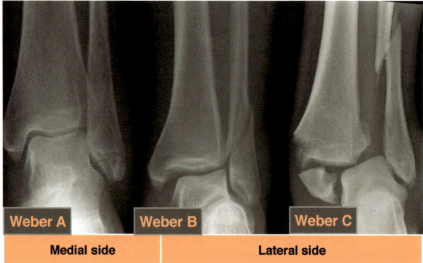

Medial side	Lateral side		
	Weber A	Weber B	Weber C
0 (no fracture or tenderness)	Conservative	Conservative	Operative
1 (medial malleolar fracture or medial side tenderness)	Operative	Operative	Operative
2 (posterior malleolus fracture)	Operative	Operative	Operative

Figure 5.10 Weber ankle fracture classification and management

INITIAL MANAGEMENT FOR CLOSED ANKLE FRACTURES

- Complete assessment checklist
- Analgesia
- Reduce fracture and secure in below knee backslab
- If isolated syndesmosis injury then image fibula head
- Check x-ray
- If fracture reduced and stable may be discharged to elevate and non-weight bear with fracture clinic follow up

ADMISSION REQUIRED IF:

- Unable to cope at home
- Unstable injury for fixation

ORTHOPAEDIC EMERGENCY: TIME TO WAKE UP THE REGISTRAR

- Talar shift that cannot be reduced in Emergency Department

Initial treatments of other common presentations

- **Trochanteric bursitis**

    Symptoms and signs: Pain over greater trochanter.

    Investigation: X-ray and bloods

    SHO management: Confirm no fracture. Analgesia
    Definitive management: Usually conservative via outpatient clinic or GP

- **Bakers cyst**

    Symptoms and signs: Painful popliteal fossa in an arthritic knee. Usually identified when patient referred for ultrasound scan to rule out DVT.

    Investigation: x-ray to demonstrate arthritis and ultrasound scan if concerned

    SHO management: Analgesia and reassure

    Definitive management: Usually conservative. Ask GP to refer to knee surgeon if they want arthritis managed with joint replacement

- **Lis-franc injury**

    Symptoms and signs: Pain in midfoot following crush or twisting injury. Excessive swelling and bruising to sole of foot

    Investigation: Identified on plain film – often subtle so look for alignment of 2nd and 3rd metatarsals

    SHO management: Admit and elevate. Consider CT scan

    Definitive management: If displaced require surgery

- **Calcaneal fracture**

    Symptoms and signs: Fall onto heels from a height; such as jumping from a window or falling from a ladder
    Investigation: x-ray ankle and AP heel

    SHO management: Check the lumbar spine. Analgesia, wool and crepe bandage (these swell profusely) and admit for elevation and further investigation. If applicable tell the patient to stop smoking.

    Definitive management: Currently controversial. Recent evidence shows that many of these will do as well managed conservatively as if they are fixed. However, if the fractures are severely displaced will need open reduction and internal fixation.

- **Talus neck fracture**

    Symptoms and signs: Pain following forced dorsiflexion. Snowboarders' fracture.

    Investigation: x-ray and CT scan

    SHO management: Admit and elevate

    Definitive management: If displaced will need fixation as high chance of avascular necrosis

Chapter 5

Further reading

Henrichs A. A review of knee dislocations. J. Athl. Train. 2004; 39 :365–9.

Kakarlapudi TK, Bickerstaff DR. Knee instability: isolated and complex.
West. J. Med. 2001; 174 :266–72.

McNamara IR, Smith TO, Shepherd KL, Clark AB, Nielsen DM, Donell S, et al. Surgical fixation methods for tibial plateau fractures. Cochrane database Syst. Rev. 2015;

SKILL STATION: REDUCTION OF ANKLE FRACTURE DISLOCATION

INDICATION
- Ankle fracture with talar shift

TEAM REQUIRED
- 1 person to plaster
- 1 person to hold thigh
- 1 person to manipulate ankle
- 1 person to monitor and provide sedation

PREPARATION
- Gain consent - ensure the patient is aware of risk of need to repeat reduction and further fracture

EQUIPMENT
- Plaster trolley
- Sedation as per hospital protocol.

Chapter 5

STEP 1: Support leg and prepare plaster

Set up equipment and ensure the patient given adequate analgesia and sedation to ensure the leg is relaxed. Have one person holding the leg under the thigh and one person ready with wool and plaster.

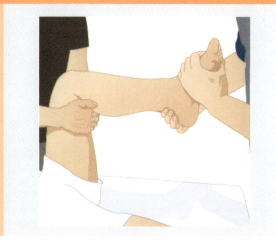

LOWER LIMB

STEP 2: Apply wool and plaster

Ask your assistant to apply a single
roll of wool from the toes to the tibial
tuberosity.

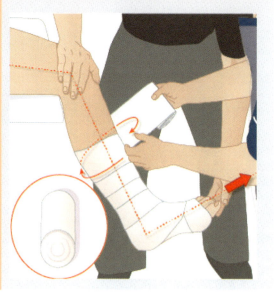

Lower Limb: Reduction of Ankle Fracture Dislocation

STEP 3: Reduce fracture

Apply the backslab and reduce the fracture. This is achieved by holding the calcaneus with the hand on the lateral side and applying pressure towards your other hand which is securing the tibia. Be mindful to keep the ankle in neutral to allow anatomical reduction – you will need to actively dorsiflex the ankle to achieve this.

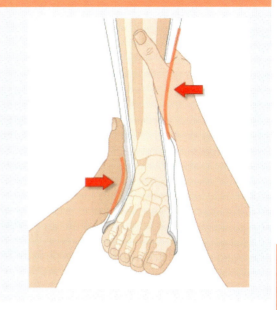

STEP 4: Elevate leg and request radiograph

Complete a tidy outer layer of crepe bandage and elevate the ankle and order a check x-ray.

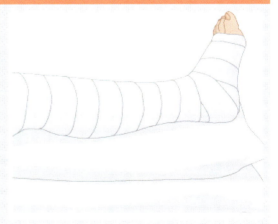

Chapter 6

Chapter 6: Orthopaedic Infections

Infections of Skin, Joints, Bones, Soft Tissue and Prostheses

Written by Andy Dekker

Chapter 6: Orthopaedic Infections Contents

1. Cellulitis	p87	4. Bursitis	p91
2. Osteomyelitis	p88	5. Periprosthetic infection	p92
3. Septic arthritis	p90		

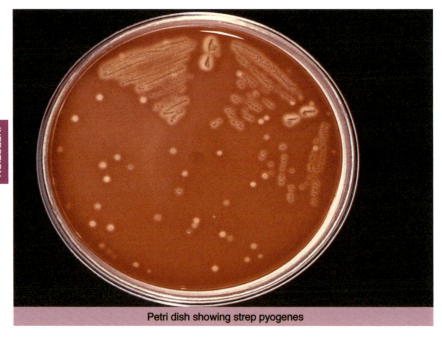

Petri dish showing strep pyogenes

Orthopaedic Infections Assessment Checklist

Infection Factors (Site)	• Location. Is there a joint involved?
Infection Factors (Side)	• Left or right
Infection Factors (Duration of onset)	• Hours, days, weeks. • Speed of spread
Infection Factors (Precipitating injury)	• Skin break or underlying fracture?
Infection Factors (Previous surgery)	• What, when and by whom?
Systemic features	• Temps and sweats • Fevers and chills
Infection Factors	• Weight bearing status
Patient Factors	• Past Medical History • Drugs and allergies • Last meal • Occupation
Examination Observation	• Rubor (red) • Calor (hot) • Dolor (pain) • Tumour (swelling)
Examination Wound	• Range of movement - Compare to other side • Discharge - Pus, serous, haemoserous • Cellulitis

Chapter 6

Other Features
- Pain on passive stretch – compartment syndrome
- Distal neurovascular involvement
- Crepitus – gas gangrene
- Rapid spread – necrotising fasciitis

Investigation
- Bloods: CRP, ESR, FBC, U&Es
- Radiographs: AP and lateral of affected area

Kocher Criteria (To help you diagnose a septic joint)

90% chance of septic arthritis if 3 out of 4 of the following are present :

- WBC > 12,000 cells/µl
- Inability to bear weight
- Fever > 101.3° F (38.5° C)
- ESR > 40 mm/h
- CRP > 2.0 (mg/dl)

Temperature > 38.5°C is the best predictor of septic arthritis followed by elevated CRP

INFECTION

3 Topics Not To Miss

1. Necrotising fasciitis
2. Compartment syndrome
3. Deep infection

1. Cellulitis

Cellulitis is a common condition and typically managed by the hospital physicians. There are however exceptions. Infections in the hand are typically managed by the orthopaedic team due to the high risk of missing flexor tendon infection and the risk of compartment syndrome.

Cellulitis or superficial infection is a condition commonly diagnosed quickly by general practitioners where oral antibiotics may quickly be started without considering the presence of deep infection and the potential for inadvertently interfering with the potential of obtaining useful specimens for microbiology.

A thorough history and examination alongside simple investigations should make the diagnosis clear. Differentials include gout, septic arthritis, postoperative infection and the rare but serious condition of necrotising fasciitis.

ADMISSION REQUIRED IF

- Tracking erythema proximally
- Rapidly spreading erythema with patient in state of septic shock: think necrotising fasciitis
- Suspicion of underlying septic arthritis or osteomyelitis

ORTHOPAEDIC EMERGENCY: TIME TO WAKE UP THE REGISTRAR

- Possibility of necrotising fasciitis
- Need for joint aspiration and you are not confident to do so
- Shocked patient requiring higher level care

Necrotising fasciitis

Necrotising fasciitis is potentially life threatening infection of the muscle fascia rather than the superficial subcutaneous tissues. It is an aggressive and rapidly progressing condition caused by streptococci, clostridia, mixed organisms including anaerobes or Methicillin-resistant Staphylococcus aureus (MRSA). Characteristic features are disproportionate pain, signs of sepsis and rapidly spreading (over hours) swelling and bullae with discharge. Gas gangrene is another rare and serious condition cause by grossly contaminated traumatic wounds. Symptoms include signs of severe sepsis and examination findings include subcutaneous emphysema which is confirmed on x-rays. The infectious organism is Clostridium perfringens which is a gram positive anaerobe. Treatment of both of these serious infections is emergency radical debridement of all affected tissues, intravenous antibiotics

INITIAL MANAGEMENT FOR CELLULITIS

- Complete assessment checklist
- Investigate with FBC, UE, CRP, ESR
- X-ray if appropriate (underlying deep infection or alternative diagnosis such as fracture or dislocation)
- Monitor vital signs including temperature
- Mark line of erythema with marker pen and date this
- Resuscitate if shocked
- Consider aspiration of joint– don't try and aspirate through cellulitic skin as you may introduce deep infection
- Reassess when investigations available
- Commence antibiotics

Chapter 6

and higher level supportive care. (ITU or HDU). Antibiotics should be guided by the local microbiology team and are usually penicillins and vancomycin. Necrotising fasciitis is a condition typically managed by plastic surgery and an urgent referral to the emergency service is necessary in all suspected cases.

If the patient is systemically well with normal observations, a low CRP, has a normal range of movement to the nearby joints without joint effusion and no tracking erythema proximally it is reasonable to treat as superficial cellulitis and treat with oral antibiotics. Commencing antibiotics as per local hospital protocol aims to treat the most likely organisms, which include group A streptococci and Staphylococcus aureus. Typical antibiotics are therefore penicillins or macrolides if penicillin allergic.

If the patient has recently had surgery and there is a wound infection or prosthesis in situ, for example post arthroplasty, deep infection should be considered. If you are unsure then senior review is appropriate.

2. Osteomyelitis

Osteomyelitis is the infection of bone. It can be caused by direct infection if the overlying tissues are damaged, such as in a diabetic foot ulcer, but can also be caused by haematogenous spread (more common in children). Diagnosis must be made definitively with biopsy but can be aided with investigations.

X-ray findings include overlying soft tissue swelling progressing to bony lysis and later a sequestrum (necrotic bone with granulation tissue) surrounded by involucrum (periosteal bone formation). Tuberculosis classically features lysis on both sides of the joint.

Infections are commonly chronic and further investigation is appropriate with MRI and surgical biopsy before starting antibiotics, unless the patient is systemically unwell and waiting for the above would significantly delay treatment. MRI is a sensitive investigation which shows associated soft tissue collections which may also require drainage. Bone scan provides useful information of disease activity.

Common organisms are S. aureus, gram-negative bacilli and group B streptococci, as well as enterobacteria and Pseudomonas aeruginosa. Antibiotic treatment may be empirically commenced after tissue samples obtained. Treatment should then be guided by organism sensitivities and on microbiology guidance.

Risk factors include IV drug abuse, diabetes, sickle cell disease (salmonella organisms) and broken skin (especially chronic ulcers, pressure sores etc).

Acute osteomyelitis may present with signs of sepsis and necessitate urgently obtaining tissue samples in order to expedite treatment.

Be aware which department typically

A* ORTHOPAEDICS

Necrotising fasciitis is a rare infection caused (usually) by Lancefield Group A Streptococcus. The infection rapidly spreads along fascial planes and needs to be debrided urgently. The LRINEC score can be used from the bloods to help with diagnosis:

1. CRP>150mgl-1 (+4 points)
2. WCC 15-25 (+1 point) 25 (2 points)
3. Hb 11-13.5 (1 point) <11(2 points)
4. Na < 135 (2 points)
5. Creatinine > 144 mmoll-1 (2 points)
6. Glucose > 18 (1 point)

A score > 6 gives is predictive of necrotising fasciitis with a sensitivity of 90% and specificity of 97%.

Infection: Osteomyelitis

manages diabetic foot infection and osteomyelitis in your hospital. Treatment is by multidisciplinary approach and new admissions may be taken under diabetic medicine, vascular surgery or plastic surgery as well as orthopaedic surgery. Initial treatment is commonly with antibiotics and consideration of the need for surgical debridement or amputation.

INITIAL MANAGEMENT FOR OSTEOMYELITIS

- Complete assessment checklist
- Investigate with FBC, UE, CRP, ESR
- X-ray
- Monitor vital signs including temperature
- Mark any surrounding erythema with marker pen and date this
- Resuscitate if shocked
- Consider aspiration of joint
- Reassess when investigations available
- Commence antibiotics if appropriate
- Consider further investigation/biopsy

ADMISSION REQUIRED IF

- Acute infection

ORTHOPAEDIC EMERGENCY: TIME TO WAKE UP THE REGISTRAR

- Patient unwell and washout required

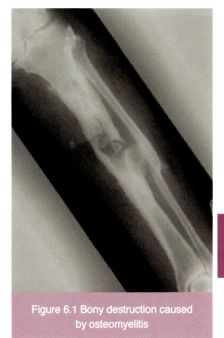

Figure 6.1 Bony destruction caused by osteomyelitis

3. Septic arthritis

Septic arthritis is the infection of a joint. It can be caused by haematogenous spread of infection or direct spread by nearby infection (osteomyelitis for example). Common joints include the knee and in children the hip. Patients at risk include the immunosuppressed, diabetics and intravenous drug users.

Causative organisms include S. aureus, streptococci, gram negative bacilli and anaerobic organisms. Differential diagnosis includes gout and osteoarthritic flare up. Diagnosis can only be proven if an organisms is isolated however in the acute setting this is a clinical diagnosis. The absence of visible organisms on gram stain or the presence of crystal arthropathy does not rule out infection. One study found the sensitivity of microscopy of joint aspiration to be 58% and fall to only 12% if the patient had already received antibiotics, which is a common occurrence as general practitioners will often treat what is suspected to be a cellulitis or superficial infection with subsequent clinical deterioration prompting urgent review by the orthopaedic service. It is alarming that isolation of an organism by culture is only positive in 79% of cases and falls to 28% if samples are taken after antibiotics administered.

Each hospital will have a local policy for the management of septic arthritis however it is typical to avoid administration of antibiotics until microbiological specimens are obtained (i.e. joint aspiration or deep tissue samples) unless the patient is suffering from severe sepsis and the delay in treatment will be to the detriment of the patient. This is clinical judgement and involvement of your registrar is essential. In the emergency setting an aspiration is usually taken and antibiotics commenced as per local microbiology protocols. If the patient is not haemodynamically unstable then ideally an open or arthroscopic washout with synovial biopsy is the preferred means for obtaining deep tissue samples and treating the infection. Antibiotics can then be commenced. Serial aspiration has been used to treat infection however is not the preferred rationale in most cases.

Treatment is by multidisciplinary approach and involvement of your local microbiologist is necessary in all cases. Further surgical washout and debridement with a prolonged course of antibiotics is often necessary.

INITIAL MANAGEMENT FOR SEPTIC ARTHRITIS

- Complete assessment checklist
- Investigate with FBC, UE, CRP, ESR
- X-ray
- Monitor vital signs including temperature
- Mark any surrounding erythema with marker pen and date this
- Resuscitate if shocked
- Consider aspiration of joint
- Reassess when investigations available
- Commence antibiotics if appropriate
- Consider need for urgent surgical washout

ADMISSION REQUIRED IF

- Essential

ORTHOPAEDIC EMERGENCY: TIME TO WAKE UP THE REGISTRAR

- Diagnosis of septic arthritis mandates admission and is an emergency

4. Bursitis

Infection of the prepatellar and olecranon bursa is common due to their superficial and exposed position. These synovial lined closed sacs function to reduce friction. A sterile inflammation can result from acute, occupational or recreational trauma, gout or pseudogout crystal deposition or systemic disease such as rheumatoid arthritis. The most common presentation of post traumatic as a result of occupation involving kneeling or heavy leaning on the elbow. Infection results from cellulitis but can also be secondary to haematogenous spread.

The causative organisms are the same as for cellulitis and septic arthritis.

Assessment should differentiate between infected and non-infected bursitis. Both will feature a fluctuant swelling over the tip of the olecranon or anterior to the patella. This is distinctly different from a joint effusion, which should not be present and if is present suggests septic arthritis. Infected cases feature raised temperature, increased temperature locally over bursa on examination and surrounding cellulitis. Infected cases are often painful whereas non infected cases are typically painless. Aspiration of pus is also diagnostic of infection.

Treatment of infected cases is antibiotics and non-steroidal anti-inflammatory analgesia in the first instance and bursal aspiration. The limb should be rested in the elevated position. Surgical incision and drainage or bursectomy should be considered in severe cases not responding to initial treatment or recurrent cases. Non infected cases do not necessitate any admission, antibiotics or further drainage. Aspiration to diagnose infection may provide symptomatic relief however the swelling may recur. The patient should be advised of this. Over time this condition is self-limiting however advice should be given to seek medical attention if signs of infection emerge.

Septic arthritis can be differentiated by the painless passive joint movement and lack of joint effusion with localised swelling anterior to the patella or over the olecranon tip.

INITIAL MANAGEMENT FOR PREPATELLA OR OLECRANON BURSITIS:

- Complete assessment checklist
- Investigate with FBC, UE, CRP, ESR
- X-ray if diagnosis unclear
- Monitor vital signs including temperature
- Mark any surrounding erythema with marker pen and date this
- Resuscitate if shocked
- Consider aspiration
- Reassess when investigations available
- Commence antibiotics if appropriate
- Consider need for surgical drainage

ADMISSION REQUIRED IF

- Infected bursitis

ORTHOPAEDIC EMERGENCY: TIME TO WAKE UP THE REGISTRAR

- Possible septic arthritis

5. Periprosthetic infection

Periprosthetic joint infection is a serious complication of arthroplasty. Risk factors include diabetes, obesity, male sex, smoking, malnutrition, alcohol excess, immunocompromised, intravenous drug abuse, nasal carriage of S.aureus, previous surgery and poor postoperative wound care. The risk is estimated at 1-2% for hip and knee surgery. Early infection can be secondary to direct seeding during implantation from skin flora or environment. Secondary haematogenous spread and recurrence of previous infection are other causes.

Prevention includes patient optimisation; all elective patients in the UK are screened preoperatively for nasal carriage of MRSA and are treated with decolonisation therapy with nasal mupirocin ointment and chlorhexidine wash if found to be positive. Nutritional status should be optimised, smoking stopped and advice on weight loss if obese. Intraoperative measures include laminar air flow, careful skin preparation, antibiotic prophylaxis, blood conservation and antibiotic impregnated cement. Body exhaust suits have also been used however have not been proven to be effective. Postoperative measures include antibiotic prophylaxis and evacuation drains to prevent haematoma.

Common causative organisms include S.aureus, Staphylococcus epidermidis, gram negative and coagulase-negative staphylococci. Methicillin-resistant S. aureus and vancomycin resistant Enterococci spp are an increasing risk.

To diagnose a periprosthetic infection definitively two positive cultures with the same organism or a communicating sinus is required. Minor diagnostic criteria include a raised CRP and ESR, raised WCC and positive histology. In the emergency department the diagnosis cannot be confirmed and you must act out of suspicion. Patients should be commenced on antibiotics immediately only if absolutely necessary (i.e. patient with severe sepsis where delay to obtain an aspirate or deep sample in theatre puts the patient at significant risk), and after discussion with your registrar. As stated above the chances of obtaining a positive culture result following the commencement of antibiotics is significantly reduced. Unfortunately a common scenario is the patient who has first been started on oral antibiotics by their general practitioner to treat a presumed superficial infection which did not settle. In this setting a positive culture may never be obtained. Clinical suspicion with an obviously deep infection macroscopically may be what guides empirical therapy on this basis.

Treatment is surgical with irrigation and debridement, and obtaining multiple deep tissue samples at the same time. The success of debridement and implant retention (DAIR) is up to 90%, however cannot be performed if the wound cannot be closed. Attempts at implant retention are often coupled with exchange of polyethylene components (reduces failure rate by up to 33%) or, for hip arthroplasty, femoral head or stem exchange. In knee arthroplasty an extensive synovectomy is often performed. The aim is to reduce the bacterial load and remove biofilm which cannot be reached by systemic antibiotics.

If an initial debridement is not successful then a two stage procedure is often indicated with an initial debridement, removal of metalwork and insertion of antibiotic impregnated spacer and a period of antibiotics (typically 6 weeks). An antibiotic-free period then follows (typically 2 weeks) where clinical response and inflammatory markers are monitored to ensure infection has been successfully treated and not simply suppressed. Following this a second stage definitive revision procedure is performed. Alternatively a single stage revision is considered reasonable if there is a known organism with an effective antibiotic option. Single stage procedure decreases morbidity however may be associated with a higher reinfection rate, although this has not been proven.

INITIAL MANAGEMENT FOR SUSPECTED PERIPROSTHETIC INFECTIONS

- Complete assessment checklist
- Investigate with FBC, UE, CRP, ESR
- X-ray
- Monitor vital signs including temperature
- Mark any surrounding erythema with marker pen and date this
- Swab wound
- Resuscitate if shocked
- Consider aspiration – must be performed in the operating theatre under sterile conditions
- Reassess when investigations available
- Commence antibiotics only if appropriate
- Consider need for surgical washout and debridement

ADMISSION REQUIRED IF

- Any possibility of deep infection

ORTHOPAEDIC EMERGENCY: TIME TO WAKE UP THE REGISTRAR

- Possible deep infection, need for aspiration in theatre

Further reading

1. Hindle P, Davidson E, Biant L. Septic arthritis of the knee: the use and effect of antibiotics prior to diagnostic aspiration. Annals of The Royal College of Surgeons of England. 2012;94(5):351-355. doi:10.1308/003588412X13171221591015.

2. Baumbach SF, Lobo CM, Badyine I, Mutschler W, Kanz KG. Prepatellar and olecranon bursitis: literature review and development of a treatment algorithm. Arch Orthop Trauma Surg. 2014 Mar;134(3):359-70. doi: 10.1007/s00402-013-1882-7.

3. Bhaveen H Kapadia, Richard A Berg, Jacqueline A Daley, Jan Fritz, Anil Bhave, Michael A Mont, Periprosthetic Joint Infection, Lancet, http://dx.doi.org/10.1016/S0140-6736(14)61798-0

Chapter 6

SKILL STATION: ASPIRATION OF A NATIVE KNEE

INDICATION	• Suspected septic arthritis of the knee
TEAM REQUIRED	• 1 person to perform aspiration • It is useful but not essential to have an assistant
PREPARATION	• Gain consent – ensure the patient is aware of risk of introducing infection
EQUIPMENT	• Chlorhexidine skin prep. 2x20ml syringes. White (21G) needle. 2x white top sterile universal containers

INFECTION

STEP 1: Prep skin

Prep the skin around the knee with the chlorhexidine. Drape around the knee to give yourself a sterile field. Ensure the toes and patella are pointing towards the ceiling.

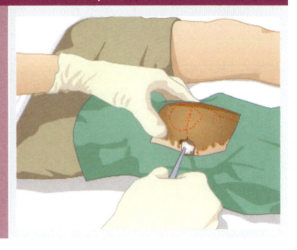

Infection: Aspiration Of A Knee

STEP 2: Aspirate joint

Palpate the patella and pull it gently laterally so that you are able to identify the gutter between the patella and the femur. Insert your needle underneath the patella in this gutter in line with the proximal pole of the patella.

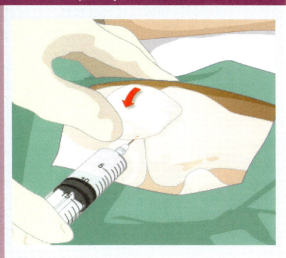

STEP 3: Send samples to microbiology

Aspirate the knee to dryness and decant a fluid sample into the universal containers. Call the microbiology technician to organise an urgent gram stain, culture and sensitivity and crystal analysis of the fluid.

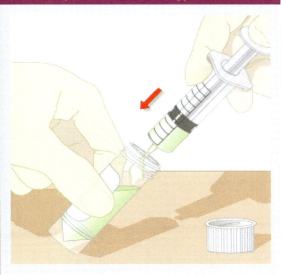

Chapter 7

Chapter 7: Spines

Back Pain, Neurology, Spinal Infections and Fractures

Chapter 7: Spines Contents

1. Back pain	p100	4. Spinal fractures	p104
2. Cauda Equina syndrome	p101	5. Cervical myelopathy	p106
3. Discitis and psoas abscess	p102	6. Other Presentations	p107

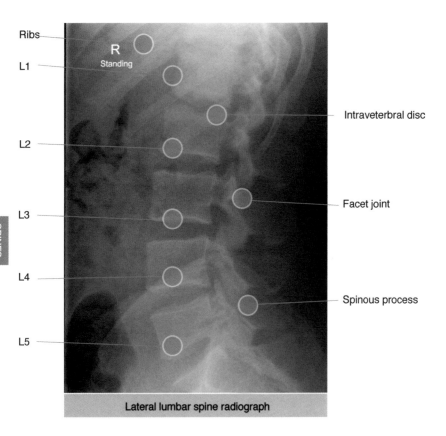

Lateral lumbar spine radiograph

Spines Assessment Checklist

History - PRESENTING FEATURES (RED FLAGS)

AGE
- <20 or >55 at first presentation

Location
- Thoracic pain

Nature
- Pain that does not improve with rest
- Night pain

Systemic features
- Fever
- Weight loss

Past medical history
- History of malignancy
- Recent trauma
- Intravenous drug use

Cauda equine compromise
- Episodes of urinary or faecal incontinence
- Not aware when bladder is full
- Not able to feel stream of urine

Examination

Look
- Deformity, swelling, curvature

Feel
- Palpate and percuss down spine and paraspinal regions

Move
- Flexion, extension, lateral rotation as able

MYOTOMES

L2	• Hip flexion
L3	• Knee extension
L4	• Ankle dorsiflexion
L5	• Extension of big toe
S1	• Ankle plantarflexion

DERMATOMES

L2	• Anterior thigh
L3	• Medial knee
L4	• Medial ankle
L5	• Lateral ankle
S1	• Sole of foot
S2	• Posterior thigh
S3 & S4	• Peri-anal (test sharp sensation)

REFLEXES

(L3/L4)	• Knee
(L4/L5)	• Ankle

DIGITAL RECTAL EXAMINATION

Tone	• Present • Absent
Squeeze power	• Good • Poor
Sensation (able to feel presence of finger)	• Present • Absent

3 Topics Not To Miss

1. Cauda equina syndrome – beware back pain with urinary symptoms
2. Psoas abscess - unusual back pain and sepsis of unknown origin
3. Cervical myelopathy – unanswered collapse query cause with upper motor neuron signs

Chapter 7

1. Back pain with or without neurology

Back pain is exceptionally common, and is associated with a significant morbidity. Often, by the time patients arrive in the Emergency Department, they have suffered with months of pain and are at the end of their tether. For this reason, patients often find it difficult to accept that initial treatment may be no more than conservative management.

Common causes of back pain include: muscular pain, osteoarthritis, disc prolapse and fracture. Uncommon causes include malignancy (often metastatic or myeloma) or infection.

The aim of your assessment is to screen for the sinister causes of back pain, including diagnoses that need to be managed urgently as an inpatient and those that can be managed as an outpatient.

As a rule of thumb, back pain with no "red flag" symptoms requires analgesia and mobilisation. They do not need admission and can be managed via the GP. Back pain with objective neurological findings warrants an MRI scan, though this could be arranged as an outpatient if the patient is able to cope at home. Back pain with red flag signs or cauda equina (see cauda equina section) requires admission and investigation.

Plain x-rays of the spine are not indicated for back pain unless there is a concern of fracture or infection. Further investigation of the back pain may be tailored for the diagnosis being considered. Urine and blood analysis are required for infection or malignancy, with serum calcium, myeloma screen and bence jones protein test for those with thoracic pain or aged over 55. CT scans to assess the stability of fractures may be required if there is significant trauma, and MRI is required when there is a concern about ligamentous stability, or disc prolapse.

INITIAL MANAGEMENT FOR BACK PAIN

- Complete assessment checklist with thorough neurological assessment
- Analgesia

ADMISSION REQUIRED IF

- Red flag symptoms identified requiring further investigation
- Objective neurology in a dermotomal/myotomal distribution
- Patient unable to cope at home

ORTHOPAEDIC EMERGENCY: TIME TO WAKE UP THE REGISTRAR

- Evidence of cauda equina syndrome (see cauda equine section)

A* ORTHOPAEDICS

A disc between two lumbar vertebra may compress the nerve root of the level below the disc, as the nerve above will have already have exited the spinal column. I.e. a L4/5 disc may compress the L5 nerve root.

SPINES

2. Cauda Equina Syndrome

The spinal cord terminates at the L1/L2 disc by dividing into multiple nerve roots. These roots take a fan-shaped appearance described as a horse's tail – the cauda equina. Importantly, within this bundle of nerves lie the roots that supply the voluntary control to the bowel and bladder. In the bladder they supply the urethral sphincter, allowing for the initiation of micturition. Also, these nerves provide sensory feedback that the bladder is filling, triggering the highly distracting sensation of the "need to pee".

If a large disc prolapse fills the space in the spinal canal and compresses these nerves, irreversible damage may occur. This needs to be decompressed, ideally within 48 hours. If this is missed, then the impact on the patient is considerable with unacceptable morbidity and has a high medico-legal implication.

The difficulty with cauda equina syndrome is that there is little consensus as to which clinical symptoms and signs will be present in each case. The most reliable findings are:

1. Urinary retention with overflow incontinence
2. Loss of trigone sensation
3. Genital numbness
4. Perianal numbness

Overflow incontinence can be established in the history by confirming if the patient is aware of their bladder filling and the "need to pee". If they are having accidents, where the patient is unaware that they have wet themselves, then you must have a high index of suspicion of cauda equina syndrome. Urinary function can be tested by performing a post void residual – a large residual indicates ineffective micturition. If you are concerned that the patient may have cauda equina syndrome then pass a urinary catheter and test the trigone sensation. This test is performed by gently tugging on the catheter. The patient will experience a sensation of needing to pass water if the trigone sensation is intact. The catheter also provides a method of reliably measuring the residual volume of the bladder and can be used to check for genital numbness.

Once admitted the patient will require an urgent MRI scan. Hospitals tend to have local protocols as to when this scan needs to occur; in the main these scans are required as soon as possible. If cauda equina syndrome is confirmed then this needs to be discussed with the spinal service or neurosurgical service (again, depending on local protocol) for consideration of urgent decompression.

INITIAL MANAGEMENT FOR CAUDA EQUINA SYNDROME

- Complete assessment checklist
- Don't forget to do a PR and trigone sensation if concerned
- Post void residual

ADMISSION REQUIRED IF

- MRI Scan required (most cases)

ORTHOPAEDIC EMERGENCY: TIME TO WAKE UP THE REGISTRAR

- Need a decision as to get a scan overnight
- MRI Scan completed and demonstrates a disc (or other lesion) causing cauda equina.

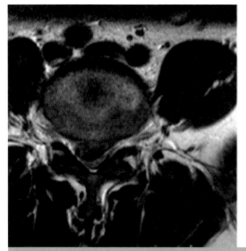 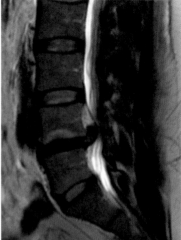

Figure 7.1 a, b Axial and sagittal T2 weighted MRI images of a broad central L4-L5 disc causing cauda equina syndrome.

3. Psoas abscess and discitis

Psoas abscess

Psoas abscess is a rare cause of hip and back pain and causes a lot of heartache as there is often poor clarity as to whether this is an "orthopaedic" or "general surgical" condition. The issue is that neither speciality particularly relishes the open surgical option of draining these abscesses. The cause is bacterial translocation from the bowel (the general surgical abscesses) or from a discitis (the orthopaedic cause).

Patients with a psoas abscess may have a relatively insidious onset of symptoms with a vague pain that is elicited by flexing and externally rotating the hip. However, they have the potential to deteriorate very rapidly and become septic. Diagnosis is usually by CT or MRI, though one unlucky F1 did manage to diagnose one when he mistook it for the femoral vein when inserting a femoral line in ITU. If possible, a sample for microbiology should be obtained before starting antibiotics and this is now completed by interventional radiology.

If the patient has signs of sepsis or septic shock, then they will require aggressive resuscitation. Initial fluid boluses should be between 10-20ml kg-1. Be prepared to involve ITU early especially if the blood pressure or heart rate fails to respond to these fluid boluses. Usually, once the abscess has been drained and antibiotics started the patient will make a recovery, though this can be slow. Be prepared for a long course of antibiotics based on local policy and culture results and check the bloods regularly to monitor response.

INITIAL MANAGEMENT FOR PSOAS ABSCESS

- Complete assessment checklist
- Check observations for evidence of sepsis.
- Sepsis 6: lactate, blood cultures, catheter, high flow O2, antibiotics ASAP (wait until cultures taken if possible), IV Fluids (with input/output monitoring)
- CT scan

> **ADMISSION REQUIRED IF**
>
> - Routine – consider discussing with general surgeons depending on local policy

> **ORTHOPAEDIC EMERGENCY: TIME TO WAKE UP THE REGISTRAR**
>
> - If patient is septic and unstable and decision needs to be made if to give antibiotics before obtaining a sample for microbiology

Discitis

Discitis is an equally rare diagnosis, and is often overlooked in patients with non-specific back pain, temperatures and raised inflammatory markers. Night pain is described as a later symptom and neurological compromise indicates severe progression of the infection.

The most common organism to cause discitis is staphylococcus aureus. However it can also be caused by escherichia coli spreading from urine tract infections, pseudomonas in intravenous drug users and salmonella in patients with sickle cell disease.

On x-ray, the following changes may be seen:

1. Narrowing of disc.
2. Loss of vertebral endplates.
3. Bony sclerosis in the vertebra above and below the affected disc.
4. Paravertebral soft tissue swelling or mass.

If these are seen or there is suspicion of discitis, then the diagnosis is confirmed with MRI scanning with gadolinium contrast.

As with psoas abscess, attempts should be made to obtain samples for culture as the antibiotic course is long. This is ideally by interventional radiology but this is not always possible. Alternatively, blood cultures may grow a causative organism, so sequential cultures may be taken (up to five times) when the patient is spiking a temperature. Antibiotics have to be prescribed according to local policy, but flucoxacillin, benzylpenicillin and rifampicin would be a good first line, empirical therapy.

If the bone or disc has been destroyed leaving an unstable spine, or if there is neurological compression or an abscess unresponsive to conservative management then open surgery is required. This will take the form of decompression, washout and stabilisation. The precise stabilisation option will depend on the site of infection and amount of destruction. Options include using pedicle screws and bars, or insertion of a cage to support the spinal column.

> **INITIAL MANAGEMENT FOR DISCITIS**
>
> - Complete assessment checklist
> - Check observations for evidence of sepsis
> - Sepsis 6: lactate, blood cultures, catheter, high flow O2, antibiotics ASAP (wait until cultures taken if possible), IV Fluids (with input/output monitoring)
> - Discuss with spinal team or neurosurgeons for need of stabilisation or biospy

> **ADMISSION REQUIRED IF**
>
> - Routine – consider discussing with general surgeons depending on local policy

Chapter 7

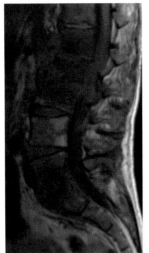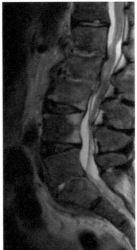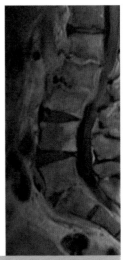

Figure 7.2 Left to right: T1, T2 and T1 post gadolinium sagittal views of L1-L2 and L2-L3 discitis. This patient was managed with IV antibiotics following blood cultures

ORTHOPAEDIC EMERGENCY: TIME TO WAKE UP THE REGISTRAR

- If patient is septic and unstable and decision needs to be made if to give antibiotics before obtaining a sample for microbiology

4. Spinal fractures

Spinal fractures come in two major groups. The first is the high-energy injuries typically seen in younger people. These may be associated with other significant injuries which may provide distraction for the patient and clinician. The other group is the low-energy injuries in the elderly, where there may be an underlying pathological process.

High energy injuries

High-energy spinal injuries are often unstable, and require a substantial index of suspicion to identify. All trauma calls, or assessment of patients with significant injuries, should include an assessment of neck and back, including a digital rectal examination to assess tone and sensation. The back is relatively fixed at the levels where the curvature changes from kyphosis to lordosis, such as C7/T1 and T12/L1. These are also areas notoriously difficult to see on plain films, so beware. If a spinal fracture is identified then CT is very useful in assessing the extent of the fracture, and in giving clues towards the stability of the fractures. MRI may be indicated if there is persistant neurology. This will identify any soft tissue disruption that may also be contrubuting to an unstable situation.

INITIAL MANAGEMENT FOR HIGH ENERGY SPINAL FRACTURES

- Complete assessment checklist
- High flow oxygen
- ABCDE and secondary survey
- Keep immobilised and on bed rest
- Analgesia and anti-emetic
- CT Scan (consider a MRI scan later to identify soft tissue injury)

Spines: Spinal Fractures

ADMISSION REQUIRED IF

- Routine for bed rest and observation

ORTHOPAEDIC EMERGENCY: TIME TO WAKE UP THE REGISTRAR

- New neurology or evidence of cauda equina syndrome

Low energy injuries

Low energy fractures occur in the elderly and are usually pathological. The disease processes that lead to these fractures include osteoporosis, primary malignancy or myeloma, metastatic disease or infection. The typical mechanism is a fall onto the bottom, with pain in the lower back that is investigated by x-ray.

On the x-ray, look to see if the fracture is a wedge or if the vertebra is crushed. Most likely the fracture will be a wedge, where the anterior cortex is compressed but the posterior cortex is intact. Lumbar wedge fractures are stable if there is an anterior height loss of less than 50%. Fractures with a height loss of more than 50%, thoracic fractures or compression/burst fractures should be admitted for further investigation. Patients with new neurology should also be admitted and cross sectional imaging obtained.

Often, patients with low energy spinal fractures will be managed conservatively. However, those with unstable spines or retropulsed fragments will need stabilisation, sometimes with decompression.

INITIAL MANAGEMENT FOR LOW ENERGY SPINAL FRACTURES

- Complete assessment checklist
- ABCDE and secondary survey
- Keep immobilised and on bed rest
- Analgesia and anti-emetic
- CT Scan (consider a MRI scan later to identify soft tissue injury)

ADMISSION REQUIRED IF

- Unstable wedge fracture (more than 50% anterior height loss)
- Burst fracture
- Thoracic fracture
- Red flag symptoms or suspicion of malignancy

ORTHOPAEDIC EMERGENCY: TIME TO WAKE UP THE REGISTRAR

- New neurology or evidence of cauda equina syndrome

A* ORTHOPAEDICS

In order to assess stability, the three column model is used.

The spine is divided into anterior (anterior percentage of vertebral body and anterior longitudinal ligament), middle (posterior percentage of vertebral body and posterior longitudinal ligament) and posterior (ligamentum flavum, facet joints and posterior ligaments). If two of the three columns are disrupted then the spine is unstable.

Chapter 7

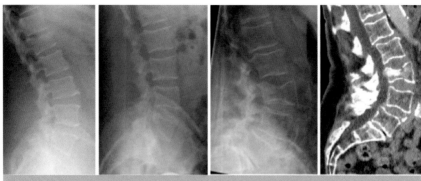

Figure 7.3 Left to right: Stable L1 wedge fracture. L1 wedge fracture with >50% loss of anterior height requiring surgical stabilisation. Burst fracture, with CT demonstrating retropulsed fragment.

5. Cervical myelopathy

A cervical myelopathy is an uncommon cause of a patient being "off legs". Most commonly these patients will be referred from the medical team who have been searching for a cause of lower limb weakness and have scanned brains to rule out a stroke, multiple blood tests for different diagnoses and finally a MRI spine is requested.

A cervical myelopathy is compression of the cord in the cervical spine. This can be from degeneration, disc or trauma and leads to a bilateral loss of function. It is an upper motor neuron lesion, so signs of increased tone, brisk reflexes and clonus may be found.

As these are delayed presentations then there is rarely any intervention required as an emergency. However, a thorough neurological examination of upper and lower limb is required as well as a detailed social history and assessment of pre-morbid state. This allows for an informed discussion about surgical options.

Unfortunately, the chance of regaining function is limited, but increasing power to the lower limbs does improve the ability for the patient to be nursed and avoid pressure sores and infection.

INITIAL MANAGEMENT FOR CERVICAL MYELOPATHY

- Complete assessment checklist
- Complete full upper and lower limb neurological examination including clonus, tone and reflexes
- Social history
- Analgesia
- Spinal surgeon opinion

ADMISSION REQUIRED IF

- Routine if not coping at home— usually these patients are already admitted

Spines: Other Presentations

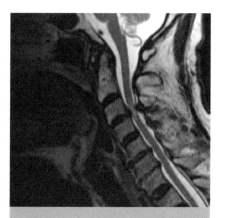

Figure 7.4 T2 weighted MRI demonstrating tight canal stenosis at C2-3. This patient was treated with a decompression

Initial treatments of other presentations

- **Facet joint dislocation**

    Symptoms and signs: Back pain with findings on x-ray or CT

    Investigation: Neurological examination followed by CT scan

    SHO management: Urgent neurosurgical or spinal opinion

    Definitive management: Reduction and stabilisation in theatre

- **Odontoid PEG (C2) Fracture**

    Symptoms and signs: Either high energy trauma in young or moderate energy trauma (e.g. fall down the stairs) in the elderly)

    Investigation: Neurological examination followed by CT scan

    SHO management: Urgent neurosurgical or spinal opinion

    Definitive management: Depends on patient and fracture factors – may be fixed or managed conservatively in a Miami or Philadelphia collar

- **Spondylolisthesis** (slip of one vertebral body away from another, may compress spinal canal)

    Symptoms and signs: Either degenerate or traumatic

    Investigation: Neurological examination followed by CT scan

    SHO management: Neurosurgical or spinal opinion if neurology, can wait overnight. Initial bed rest

    Definitive management: Depends on patient and amount of slip– may be fixed or managed conservatively

Further reading

1,. National Institute for Health and Care Excellence. Low back pain CG88. 2009.

2. Gardner A, Gardner E, Morley T. Cauda equina syndrome: a review of the current clinical and medico-legal position. Eur. Spine J. 2011; 20 :690–7.

Chapter 8

Chapter 8: Neck of Femur Fractures
Hip Fractures and Care of The Elderly

Neck of Femur Fractures Chapter Contents

1. Intracapsular fractures — p112
2. Extracapsular fractures — p113
3. Subtrochanteric fractures — p114
4. Pathological fractures — p115
5. Other Presentations — p116

Labels on AP right hip radiograph:
- Intact trabaculae
- Greater trochanter
- Intratrochanteric line
- Shentons line
- Femoral head
- Superior pubic rami
- Inferior pubic rami
- Lesser trochanter

AP right hip radiograph

NOF

108

Neck of Femur Fracture Assessment Checklist

History - PRESENTING FEATURE

Age & Time of Injury	• Delay to seek help?
Mechanism	• Mechanical fall? • Preceding symptoms? • Witnessed fall?
Past medical history	• Diagnoses • Medications • Allergies • Previous malignancy
Drug history	• Antihypertensives (hold) • Anticoagulants (check INR) • Diabetes (hold metformin / gliclazide)
Social	• Mobility (independent, one stick, two sticks, frame, wheelchair bound) • Home situation
System Review	• GI: appetite / bowel function • Respiratory: cough / shortness of breath • GUM: dysuria • Night pain or pain before falling
Cognitive	• (AMTS)

Chapter 8

Examination

OBSERVATION	• Wounds or ulcers on the leg • Leg shortening • Neurovascular status
RESPIRATORY	• Air entry • Added sounds • Chest x-ray
CARDIOVASCULAR	• Added sounds • ECG
ABDOMINAL	• Masses • Tenderness • Urine dip

Investigations

- **Bloods:** FBC, U&E, LFT, Ca2+, TFT, group and save
- **Imaging:** CXR, AP Pelvis and lateral hip
- ECG
- Urine dip

Neck of Femur Fractures

If the fracture isn't obvious on plain film radiographs
- MRI or CT if suspicion of occult fracture

Proforma
- Most hospitals have a hip fracture pro-forma that should be completed. This covers all of the checklist and ensures that hospitals gain funding for meeting the admission criteria

3 Topics Not To Miss

1. Neck of femur fracture in the young (<55 years)
2. Associated other injuries
3. Pathological fractures

Neck of femur fractures make up a significant proportion of an orthopaedic take. There are over 50,000 hip fractures each year in the United Kingdom, and this number is set to increase as the population ages. For people who sustain a neck of femur fracture, 20-30% will die within 1 year of fracture and 30% will have a significant decrease in function.

Neck of femur fractures contribute to 87% of fragility fractures and represent a state of "bone failure", much like cardiac or respiratory failure. These patients are often complex with multiple co-morbidities and medical issues which stacks against them obtaining good outcomes. Patients with hip fractures should be managed in a coordinated multidisciplinary team, with orthopaedic surgeons assessing and ensuring rapid access to surgery and Ortho-geriatric care to help optimise peri-operative medical conditions.

Guides to best practice can be found from NICE and the British Geriatric Society, and have been combined to form the UK Best Practice Tariff. This is a reward system to promote best care within hospitals, and requires that patients with a neck of femur fracture should have their operation within 36 hours, and be cared for with joint-care with an Ortho-geriatrician who provides post-operative management within a multidisciplinary team including secondary prevention for future fragility fractures.

The orthopaedic evaluation of patients with neck of femur fractures evolves around identifying the fracture pattern, as well as completing a basic assessment of the patient's medical needs that can built on by the multi-disciplinary team. The assessment checklist highlights important questions to evaluate this, and to establish the cause of fall – remember that the fracture may also have a myocardial infarction or severe sepsis which will need to be managed in priority to the broken hip!

Hip fractures are common in the elderly, and should be considered in any patient who has sustained a fall and subsequently develops hip pain. For some patients with a hip fracture, the initial x-ray will not reveal the fracture. The most sensitive tool for diagnosing a fracture in this group is a MRI scan, though CT scan may be used if a MRI is not available.

Chapter 8

1. Intracapsular fractures

An intracapsular fracture has a fracture line that runs within the capsule of the hip. This capsule is attached to the intratrochanteric line and is of critical significance. These fractures can be divided into subcaptital (just under the head), trans cervical (mid portion of neck) and basicervical (at the junction between neck and trochanters). Basicervical fractures are uncommon, and are unusual intracapsular fractures as they may be fixed like a extracapsular fracture with a dynamic hip screw and de-rotation screw.

The importance of this fracture pattern is that the blood supply to the femoral head may be compromised. The blood vessels travel in a retrograde fashion from branches of the circumflex arteries. These start at the level of the trochanters and provide a network of smaller arteries that travel up the neck to the head. If there is a fracture, these smaller arteries may be severed or kinked. This will result in subsequent avascular necrosis of the femoral head and a painful joint in a high number of cases. The treatment decision for intracapsular neck of femur fractures depends on the amount of displacement and on the patients' medical comorbidities and mobility. The greater the displacement the higher the chance of avascular necrosis if the hip is reduced and fixed with screws or a dynamic hip screw. However, the best articulating hip is the patient's own hip, so
if the fracture is not displaced and the patient is a good candidate for surgery, fixation may be offered in preference to replacement. The patient will be counselled about the potential for requiring a hip replacement in the future.

For displaced fractures and older patients, a single operation strategy is preferable. This can be with a hemiarthroplasty (replacing the hip stem and ball but leaving the acetabulum) or with a total hip replacement. A total hip replacement

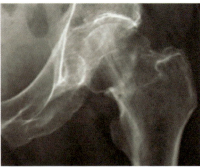
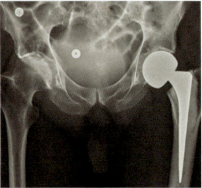

Figure 8.1 a, b Intracapsular neck of femur fracture, treated with hemiarthroplasty

has the advantage of greater longevity and improved functional outcomes, but comes at a cost of a longer operation and higher dislocation risk. Current guidance from the National Institute for Care and Clinical Excellence states that total hip replacements should be considered for patients who normally mobilise independently outdoors or use only one stick, who have no evidence of dementia and are medically fit for an anaesthetic. A good method of screening for this is to ask the patient if they can do their own shopping

INITIAL MANAGEMENT FOR INTRACAPSULAR FRACTURE

- Complete assessment checklist
- Analgesia
- Fascia iliaca block

and calculate an abbreviated mental state examination score (AMTS).

ADMISSION REQUIRED IF
- All cases

ORTHOPAEDIC EMERGENCY: TIME TO WAKE UP THE REGISTRAR
- 1. Fracture in a young patient

2. Extracapsular fractures

Extracapsular fractures are fractures that occur outside of the capsule. This means that the blood supply to the head should be intact, so the bone can be fixed rather than replaced. Initial management is identical to an intracapsular fracture, but the treatment options are different. Surgical treatment options are either a dynamic hip screw (DHS) or cephalomedullary nail.

For a "stable" intratrochanteric fracture, i.e. one that is two or three parts and the fracture line extends perpendicular to the axis of the neck; a dynamic hip screw is the treatment of choice. This implant uses a large single screw into the head that can slide in the barrel of the plate. As the patient walks, their weight promotes the fracture to collapse and compress encouraging fracture healing.

An "unstable" fracture may be involve 3 or more parts. Features that make an unstable intratrochanteric fracture include fragmentation of the greater trochanter or a four part fracture. The greater trochanter acts as the lateral buttress for any fixation and a 4 part fracture will have the lesser trochanter fractured and displaced. There is some debate as to the ideal method of fixing these fractures. The general U.K. consensus is to use a dynamic hip screw wherever possible as there is a lower reoperation rate. It is also a much cheaper implant than an intramedullary nail.

Notable exceptions to this rationale include the reverse oblique fracture, where the fracture line extends parallel to the neck of the femur. These fractures are very unstable and do badly if fixed with a dynamic hip screw. These fractures are treated with a nail.

INITIAL MANAGEMENT FOR EXTRACAPSULAR FRACTURE
- Complete assessment checklist
- Analgesia
- Fascia iliaca block

ADMISSION REQUIRED IF
- All cases

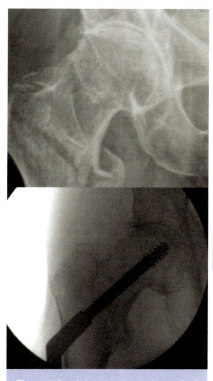

Figure 8.2 a, b Intratrochanteric neck of femur fracture, treated with dynamic hip screw

3. Subtrochanteric fractures

Subtrochanteric fractures occur up to 5cm distal to the lesser trochanter of the hip and are significant injuries. A subtrochanteric fracture has a similar bleeding potential to a diaphyseal femoral fracture and resuscitation should be prompt and comprehensive. A Thomas splint may be required to control the fracture and provide a temporary splint to reduce blood loss and provide analgesia. However place a fascia iliaca or femoral nerve block before moving the leg into the splint. Details on how to apply a Thomas splint can be found in the paediatrics section of this book in the skill station.

As these fractures are very unstable, operative management is with an intramedullary nail that spans the fracture and is locked proximally into the femoral neck and distally.

INITIAL MANAGEMENT FOR SUBTROCHANTERIC FRACTURE

- Complete assessment checklist
- Analgesia
- Fascia iliaca or femoral nerve block
- Consider Thomas splint

ADMISSION REQUIRED IF

- All cases

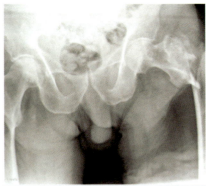

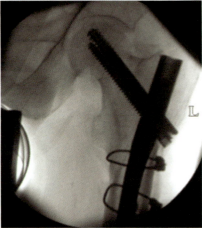

Figure 8.3 a, b Reverse oblique fracture of the left neck of femur, treated with cephalomedullary nail and cables

4. Pathological fractures

In the assessment checklist there are several questions to ask in the history to exclude a pathological fracture. Pathological fractures can come in many forms. The most common is osteoporosis, which is covered in some detail in the Ortho-geriatrics section. The next important source of pathological fractures is malignancy, which has a significant impact in the management of patients with neck of femur fractures.

Metastatic spread to bone is common in prostate, breast, lung, renal and thyroid tumours. Prostate cancer leads to sclerotic lesions in the bone, whereas thyroid and renal tumours tend to lead to lytic lesions. These pathological lesions may be detected before a fracture occurs due to pain and a decision made as to whether or not to prophylactically splint these fractures, usually with a nail.

Other tumours or malignancies that can lead to pathological fractures include multiple myeloma and primary bone tumours. Primary bone tumours pose a particular issue, as attempting to fix through these lesions may seed and spread the cancer to distal sites leading to poorer outcomes. For this reason you need to be relatively confident in your diagnosis of the primary site, and this may require additional imaging with CT chest, abdomen and pelvis alongside a thorough systems review.

Alternative causes of pathological fractures are metabolic in nature, and include the transverse stress fractures of bisphosphonates. Bisphosphonates act by inhibiting the osteolytic action of the osteoclasts. This is excellent in preventing bone resorption and reducing the overall risk of fracture in osteoporosis. However, it also prevents the normal remodelling in response to loading and stress. It is thought that repeated small stress fractures accumulate and can result in a significant low energy fracture. Further metabolic disorders that may lead to pathological fractures includes Paget's disease and hyperparathyroid.

ADMISSION REQUIRED IF

- All cases

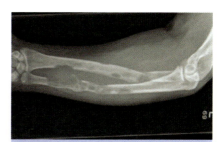

Figure 8.4 Pathological fractures are not limited to the hip, this is a pathological fracture of radius and ulna from myeloma

A* ORTHOPAEDICS

The decision to fix a pathological lesion is based on the Mirels score. This gives an indication as to how impeding a fracture might be. A score of 9 or more should be fixed

	1	2	3
Site	Arm	Leg	Hip
Lesion	Sclerotic	Mixed	Lytic
Pain	Mild	Moderate	Severe
Size	<33%	33-66%	>66%

INITIAL MANAGEMENT FOR PATHOLOGICAL FRACTURE

- Complete assessment checklist
- Analgesia
- Fascia iliaca or femoral nerve block
- Identify primary – from history or further investigations
- Bloods for FBC, U&E, LFT, Ca2+, myeloma screen
- Urine for Bence Jones protein

Chapter 8

Initial treatments of other presentations

- **Diaphyseal fractures (fragility fracture)**

    Symptoms and signs: Pain following fall or twisting injury

    Investigation: x-ray

    SHO management: Admit, Thomas splint or skin traction

    Definitive management: IM Nail

- **Distal femoral fracture (fragility fracture)**

    Symptoms and signs: Pain following fall or slip onto knees

    Investigation: X-ray, CT to define if fracture extends between the condyles

    SHO management: Admit, Thomas splint or skin traction

    Definitive management: May be treated in plaster or with a plate or IM nail.

Further reading

1. Godoy Monzon D, Iserson K V, Vazquez JA. Single fascia iliaca compartment block for post-hip fracture pain relief. J. Emerg. Med. 2007; 32 :257–62.

2. Parker M, Johansen A. Hip fracture. BMJ Br. Med. J. 2006; 333 :27–30.

3. National Institute for Health and Clinical Excellence. Hip fracture: The management of hip fracture in adults (CG 124). 2011.

SKILL STATION: FASCIA ILIACA COMPARTMENT BLOCK

INDICATION	• Intracapsular or Extracapsular neck of femur fractures
TEAM REQUIRED	• 1 person to administer block
PREPARATION	• Gain consent – ensure the patient is aware of risk of infection and of haematoma formation
EQUIPMENT	• Skin marker pen. Chlorhexidine skin prep. 5ml syringe with 5ml 1% lignocaine. 20ml syringe with blunt needle and 20-30ml long acting anaesthetic.

STEP 1: Identify landmarks

Mark landmarks: Anterior superior iliac spine (ASIS), pubic tubercle and femoral artery. Identify a point 1/3 along the line from ASIS to tubercle and mark the injection side 2cm below this point.

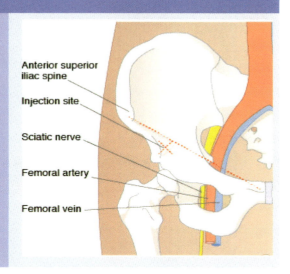

STEP 2: Prep skin

Clean the skin with chlorhexidine and inject 3-5ml of 1% lignocaine as a subcutaneous bleb at the injection site.

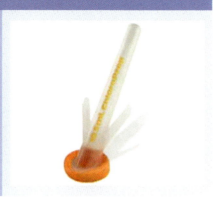

Neck of Femur Fractures: Fascia Iliaca Compartment Block

STEP 3: Insert needle

Insert a blunt needle through the skin at the injection site. The angle of the needle should be initially 90° to get through the skin, then reduce the angle to 30° to pass through the fascial layers.

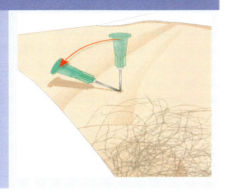

STEP 4: Advance through tissues

Advance the needle through the fascia lata (the first pop) and then through the fascia iliaca (the second pop). These pops are quite distinctive. Inject 20-30ml of long acting local anaesthetic such as 0.25% bupivacaine. This should pass easily down the needle to bathe the femoral nerve, obturator nerve and lateral cutaneous nerve of the thigh to produce the analgesic effect.

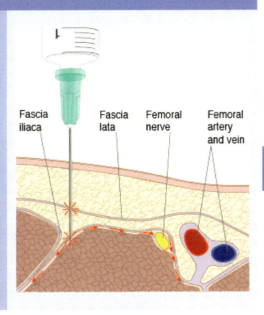

Chapter 9

Chapter 9: Paediatrics

Fractures, Injuries and Infections in Children

Chapter 9: Paediatrics Contents

1. Supracondylar fractures	p123	4. Femoral fractures	p129
2. The limping child	p125	5. Non accidental injury	p130
3. Growth plate injury	p128	6. Other Presentations	p131

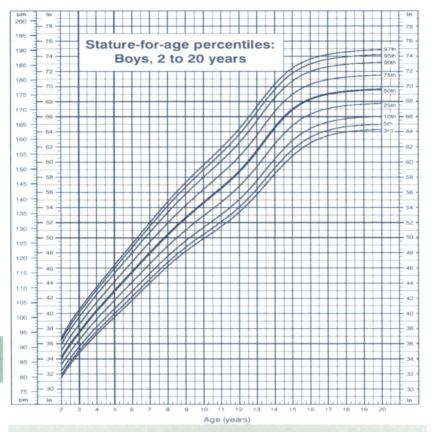

Paediatric growth chart

Paediatric Assessment Checklist
History - Presenting Feature

Age & Time of Injury	• Delay to seek help?
Mechanism	• How injury sustained • Plausible story? • Consistent story?
Past medical history	• Diagnoses • Medications • Allergies • Vaccinations • Birth (method and at term)?
Development	• Ambulatory status (sitting, crawling, walking) • Developmental milestones
System Review	• Previous injuries • ED attendances • Fever / sweats • Night pain • Appetite

*remember children are often poor historians, so consider atypical causes for any presentation such as UTI, spine or abdominal causes for pain.

Chapter 9

Examination

Observation	• Use of limbs • Affect • Interaction with parents • Parents interaction with each other
Injury	• Deformity • Pain
Associated injuries	• Wounds • Other fractures • Open fracture • Bruising

Other - Gait

Neurovascular status	• Pulses • Capillary refill time • Sensation • Function

1 Topic Not To Miss

Non accidental injury

1. Supracondylar fracture

Supracondylar fractures of the elbow are fractures that cause anxiety in even the most experienced orthopaedic surgeon. They are very common, and if your rotation occurs in the summer months, then you will almost certainly encounter a very tearful child who has fallen off the trampoline, or rather taken an ungraceful tumble from the monkey bars.

Un-displaced fractures are treated conservatively, usually by accident and emergency. The preferred management is with a collar and cuff to encourage the child to keep the elbow flexed, though sometimes an above elbow back slab is used. More substantial fractures where the distal fragment is rotated or completely displaced require surgical management.

A* ORTHOPAEDICS

The Gartland classification is used to describe supracondylar elbow fractures. This classification requires a lateral view of the elbow.

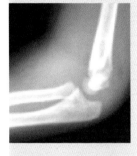

1. Minimally displaced

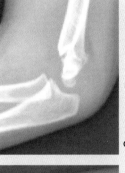

2. Displaced but posterior hinge intact. Divided into 2a (no rotation) and 2b (rotation in coronal plane seen on ap image)

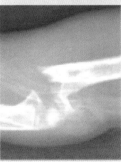

3. Off-ended

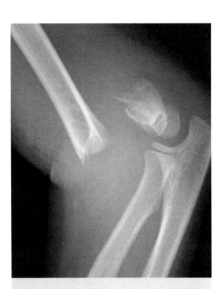

Figure 9.1 Displaced Supracondylar fracture

Chapter 9

When examining these patients, careful assessment of neurovascular status is vital. The median nerve and brachial artery run along the humerus at almost the exact point at which a supracondylar fracture occurs. These nerves may be injured in this fracture. It is the anterior interosseous nerve that is most commonly involved (essential for flexing the interphalangeal joint of the thumb when making an "ok" sign).

In order of urgency, a displaced supracondylar fracture may feature:

Cold hand, no pulses

A cold hand with no pulses suggests the artery is caught in the fracture site. The forearm will soon develop ischaemia. Splint the arm in a position of comfort (do not fully flex as this may further compromise vascular function) and prep for theatre for manipulation under anaesthesia plus k-wire stabilisation as an emergency. Remind your registrar to alert the vascular surgeons as they may be required to explore the artery during the operation.

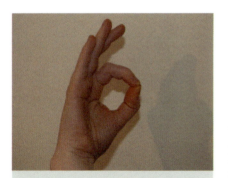

Figure 9.1 OK sign for testing AIN. (AIN supplies flexor hallux longus muscle)

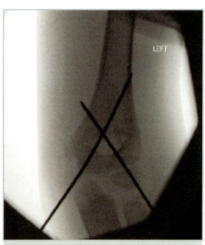

Figure 9.2 Intra-operative image of crossed k-wire fixation for supracondylar fracture

Warm hand, no pulses or neurological impairment

The warm hand without pulses phenomenon is thought to be due to brachial artery vasospasm. Discuss this patient with your registrar and prep for theatre as most would want to operate on this overnight to minimise trauma to the nerves and blood vessels.

Warm hand, pulses, no neurovascular deficit

While this eventuality can potentially wait overnight and be done on a planned trauma list, discuss this with the registrar as manipulating this acutely is much easier than in the morning when the swelling has taken hold.

There is much debate as to the best method for fixing these fractures. Broadly, k-wire fixation can use 2 or 3 wires in a crossed configuration (medial and lateral entry) or lateral only entry, diverging to provide stability. Lateral wires reduce the risk of ulna nerve damage, but need to be carefully placed to gain sufficient stability of the distal fragment.

INITIAL MANAGEMENT FOR SUPRACONDYLAR FRACTURE

- Complete assessment checklist
- Analgesia
- AP and lateral x-ray
- Collar and cuff or backslab
- Assess neurovascular status – especially hand warmth, pulses and AIN ("OK" sign)

ADMISSION REQUIRED IF

- Displaced fracture for theatre

ORTHOPAEDIC EMERGENCY: TIME TO WAKE UP THE REGISTRAR

- Cold hand
- AIN ("OK" sign) or other nerve dysfunction
- Pulses absent

2. The limping child

Children with a limp are a common presentation to GPs, the emergency department or paediatric admissions and cause another great source of worry. While most patients have benign causes for limping, you must not miss a sinister cause as it will have catastrophic consequences for the child and family.

The causes of hip (and knee) pain in children that need to be excluded are:

- Septic arthritis (all ages)
- Slipped upper femoral epiphysis (boys 13-15 girls 11-13 approx)
- Perthes disease (age 4-8 approx)
- Trauma (all ages)
- Transient synovitis (reactive arthritis)

Septic arthritis is an orthopaedic emergency and needs to be identified and managed rapidly. For this reason every child referred with a limp should have a full set of observations and blood tests for inflammatory markers and white cells. Septic arthritis is covered in more detail in the infections chapter.

A* ORTHOPAEDICS

Kocher's criteria can be used to try and predict the chance of a limp in a child being due to septic arthritis and is a trauma meeting favourite:

1. Temperature >38.5°C
2. White cell count > 12,000 cellsµL-1
3. ESR> 40mmh-1 (alternatively CRP>20mgL-1)
4. Child unable to weight bear

The likelihood of septic arthritis if 4/4 are present is 99%, 3/4 93%, 2/4 40% and 1/4 3%

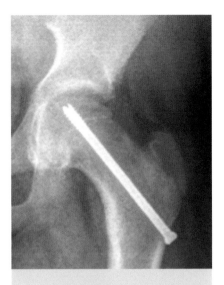

Figure 9.3 SUFE fixed with percutaneous screws

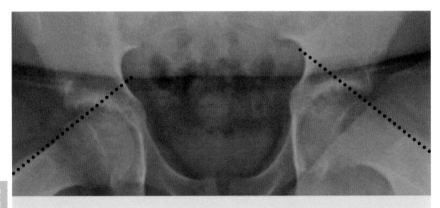

Figure 9.4 Importance of a frog leg lateral, this subtle left sided slip was not apparent on the AP view. Note how a line drawn on the superior neck does not transect the femoral head on the left hip (Klein's line). This is treated with a screw to prevent further slip (right image)

Slipped upper femoral epiphysis (SUFE)

Slipped upper femoral epiphysis (SUFE) occurs stereotypically on overweight adolescent boys, though may present in any child with a limp. These injuries are sheering fractures through the growth plate and may be acute or chronic, stable or unstable. You will usually be investigating acute (less than 3 weeks duration), unstable (unable to weight bear, even with a crutch) slips. To diagnose a SUFE a frog-leg lateral view is required in addition to the standard AP pelvis x-ray. X-ray signs may be subtle, if concerned then ask for senior support and keep the child on bed rest for observation.

Perthes disease is a type of avascular necrosis of the femoral head. It is thought to be due to a disruption of the blood supply as the anatomy of the femur changes during normal growth, but the exact cause is unknown. If you are lucky (and the patient unlucky) then x-ray changes may be apparent with a flattened femoral head, bone cysts and joint space widening with effusion. However, in many cases initial x-ray images will be normal. Diagnosis is frequently obtained by admitting the patient overnight on bed rest. If the limp fails to respond to simple analgesia then further imaging, such as a MRI, is required.

Trauma is a cause of limp that may act as a red herring, as it is possible to have infection, SUFE or perthes in addition to trauma, so maintain your guard. If in doubt, admit the patient for bed rest, give analgesia and review to ensure the limp has improved before discharging.

Transient synovitis is a final cause of limp, a diagnosis of exclusion. The synovitis is usually preceded by an infection, such as a sore throat or common cold. The joint is irritable and inflammatory markers may be raised due to underlying minor infection. This condition is self-limiting and improves with simple analgesia, but children need to be fully worked up for other causes of limp before deciding on this diagnosis.

INITIAL MANAGEMENT FOR LIMPING CHILDREN

- Complete assessment checklist
- Analgesia
- Examine knee, hip and spine
- Bloods for inflammatory markers
- X-ray pelvis (and knee if painful) AP and frog leg lateral
- Observe for analgesia effect
- Bed rest
- Consider ultrasound guided aspiration if suspicious of infection or MRI

ADMISSION REQUIRED IF

- Not unreasonable in all cases for observation
- Evidence of infection or SUFE
- Further investigation

ORTHOPAEDIC EMERGENCY: TIME TO WAKE UP THE REGISTRAR

- Evidence of infection

Chapter 9

3. Growth plate injuries

Fractures through the growth plate occur while children are skeletally immature. Unlike adult bones which are more brittle, children's bones are more elastic and fail through bending (plastic deformation or buckle fracture) or by fracturing through the relatively weak hypertrophic zone in the growth plate.

The classification of growth plate injuries gives an indication of the amount of energy applied to create the fracture, and by the probability of future growth abnormalities.

- Salter Harris 1 fractures are rare and are fractures straight through the growth plate.
- Salter Harris 2 fractures have a fracture line that runs through the growth plate and exits through the metaphysis. These are the most common growth plate injury and are seen frequently in adolescent fractures of the distal radius.
- Salter Harris 3 fractures occur when the fracture extends through the growth plate and exits through the epiphysis – often through the articular surface.
- Salter Harris 4 fractures have a fracture line that extends from the metaphysis through the growth plate and exits via the epiphysis
- Salter Harris 5 fractures are very rare and are crush fractures to the growth plates and have a high chance of causing growth arrest.

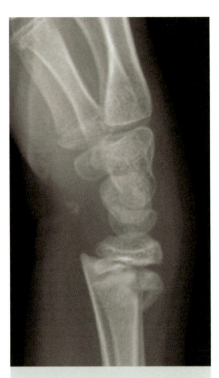

Figure 9.5 Salter Harris 2 fracture distal radius

If you are referred a patient with a growth plate injury then the first priority should be to splint it in a backslab for pain relief. Many minimally displaced fractures can be treated conservatively, some with a gentle tweak in the emergency department to reduce the fracture. Others will need a manipulation in theatre dependant on degree of deformity and patients' age.

 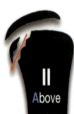 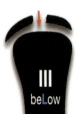 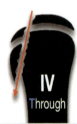 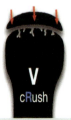

Figure 9.6 Salter Harris Classification: remembered by the mnemonic SALTR

INITIAL MANAGEMENT FOR GROWTH PLATE INJURY

- Complete assessment checklist
- Analgesia
- Check neurovascular status
- Splint in backslab
- Check x-ray

ADMISSION REQUIRED IF

- Manipulation required in theatre
- Concern about NAI

ORTHOPAEDIC EMERGENCY: TIME TO WAKE UP THE REGISTRAR

- Neurovascular deficit
- Open fracture

4. Femoral fractures

Femoral fractures in children are usually caused by significant twisting injuries. These fractures often look very dramatic, but can often be managed conservatively, depending on the age of the patient.

In the very young (< 6 months), virtually all femoral fractures can be treated conservatively with a brace (a pavlick harness) or a spica cast. These will need to be arranged during daylight hours, so it would not be unreasonable to put the child in traction (gallows traction) overnight.

The young child (7 months – 5 years) will need to be managed depending on the amount of shortening on the x-ray. For those with less than 2cm shortening, a spica cast is the treatment of choice. If the femur is shortened by more than 2 cm then the patient can still have a plaster, though usually after a period of traction on the ward to restore the length. Alternatively the fracture can be fixed in theatre with either a plate or with flexible intramedullary nails. For the older child (6-11 years) the parents will struggle to manage the child in a spica cast. While not impossible, these children will often be stabilised in theatre with flexible nails to control the fracture while it heals. Children approaching skeletal maturity (>11 years) will also require operative stabilisation, though this is usually by plate fixation or rigid intramedullary nail.

In the initial phase, all these children may be managed with traction. This fracture indicates a significant force, so complete a thorough secondary survey as there may be associated injuries. Remember to pay careful attention to the history, especially if in a toddler or younger, as these fractures are the second most common fracture caused by non-accidental injury.

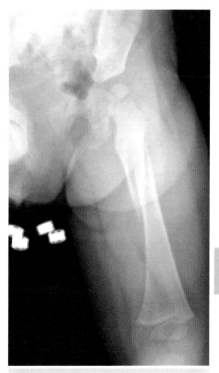

Figure 9.7 Right spiral mid-shaft femoral fracture

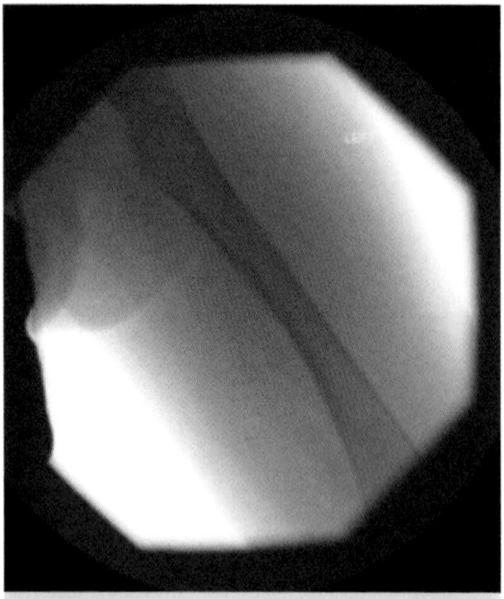

Chapter 9

Figure 9.8 Femoral shaft fracture in an infant. This was left in traction for 3 days then placed in a hip spica in theatre

INITIAL MANAGEMENT FOR FEMORAL FRACTURE

- Complete assessment checklist
- Analgesia
- Splint in Thomas splint
- Check x-ray

ADMISSION REQUIRED IF

- Will be required to schedule definitive management – spica cast or theatre
- Suspicion of NAI

ORTHOPAEDIC EMERGENCY: TIME TO WAKE UP THE REGISTRAR

- Open fracture

5. Non accidental injury (NAI)

It is a sad fact of modern life that children will be abused. Every few years a horror story will hit national press, invariably culminating from the death of a child at the hand of those who were supposed to be looking after it. This may be parents, family or carers, your job is to keep an open mind.

The recurring learning point from child protection disasters are the missed opportunities where the child presents to multiple agencies with injuries or signs of abuse. As front-line orthopaedics, you are in an excellent position to be the first to sound the alarm. However, to do this you must consider non-accidental causes as a potential mechanism for any injury in a child.

Features in the story that should cause significant concern are:

- Vague or inconsistent history
- Implausible mechanism of injury - is the child mobile? Could the proposed mechanism have caused that injury?
- Delay in seeking medical attention
- Unusual patient behaviour
- Repeated attendances at the emergency department
- Evidence of multiple healing fractures on x-ray (periosteal reactions)

If you have concerns, admit the patient. Alert your seniors and discuss with the paediatric team. Though time consuming, innocent parents usually understand the need for investigation and are prepared to wait as they want the best care for their child.

INITIAL MANAGEMENT FOR SUSPECTED NON ACCIDENTAL INJURY

- Complete assessment checklist
- Analgesia
- Manage injury
- Careful and thorough documentation of history given
- Refer to paediatric / child protection team for further assessment / skeletal survey etc.

ADMISSION REQUIRED IF

- For all patients

ORTHOPAEDIC EMERGENCY: TIME TO WAKE UP THE REGISTRAR

- Life or limb threatening injury
- Most can be admitted as usual, flagged up to the paediatric team and managed in the morning

Initial treatments of other presentations

- **Congenital dislocation of hip**

Symptoms and signs: Screened for at birth – hip dislocates when adducted and axial loading (Barlow test) or clunks and reduces on flexion and abduction (Ortolani test)

Investigation: Outpatient ultrasound

SHO management: Refer to paediatric outpatient clinic

Definitive management: Pavlik harness or hip spica

- **Elbow fracture (not supracondylar**

Symptoms and signs: Painful swollen elbow following injury

Investigation: X-ray

SHO management: Backslab and admit

Definitive management: Depends on fracture: medial or lateral epicondyle fracture may need fixing and displaced radial neck fractures need theatre for manipulation

- **Forearm fractures (both bones)**

Symptoms and signs: Painful, deformed forearm following injury

Investigation: X-ray

SHO management: Backslab and admit

Definitive management: May remodel but often needs manipulation

- **Toddler fracture**

Symptoms and signs: Painful lower leg in an infant, may present as just non weight bearing

Investigation: X-ray – fracture may not be apparent

SHO management: Can have a full cast and review in fracture clinic

Definitive management: Conservative

Further reading

1. National Institute for Health and Care Excellence. CG 89: When to suspect child maltreatment. 2009.
2. Badkoobehi H, Choi PD, Bae DS, Skaggs DL. Management of the pulseless pediatric supracondylar humeral fracture. J. Bone Joint Surg. Am. 2015; 97 :937–43.
3. Perry DC, Bruce C. Evaluating the child who presents with an acute limp. BMJ. 2010; 341 :c4250–c4250.

SKILL STATION: APPLICATION OF THOMAS SPLINT

INDICATION	• Diaphyseal femoral fracture
TEAM REQUIRED	• 1 person to apply skin traction and place Thomas splint • 1 person to hold thigh • 1 person to maintain in-line traction
PREPARATION	• Give plenty of analgesia and apply foam straps to Thomas splint

Paediatrics: Application Of A Thomas Splint

STEP 1: Measure leg

Measure the patient's leg length and thigh circumference. A ring should be selected that is 4cm larger than the thigh to permit swelling. 20cm should be added to the length of the leg to set the splint.

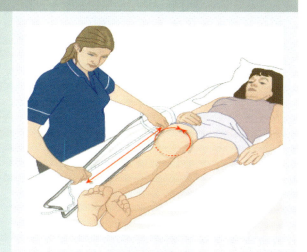

STEP 2: Apply traction strap

Apply the traction strip to the leg with the foam padding over the malleoli and a hand breath gap between the end of the strip and the sole of the foot. Secure the strip with bandage to the level of the fracture, leaving the knee and ankle exposed.

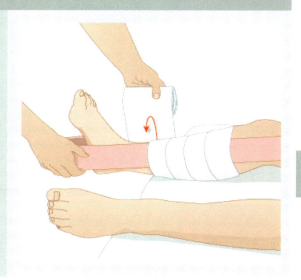

Chapter 9

STEP 3: Secure splint beneath leg

With in-line traction being applied to the ankle and the thigh being supported, the splint is inserted under the leg.

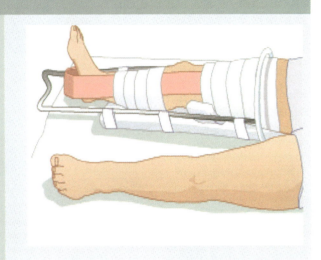

STEP 4: Apply and tension cord

Loop the cord around the frame – the lateral length goes over the bar and the medial cord goes under. Tie the cord with windlass (often 2 lollypop sticks) and twist the windlass to obtain tension in the cord.

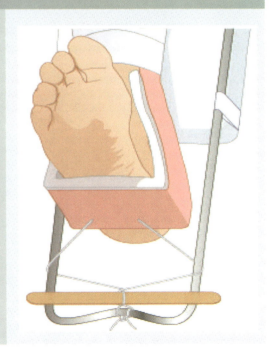

STEP 5: Apply traction

If available then the splint should be balanced with weights and pulleys. However, if not then the tension of the cord around the windlass will maintain traction.

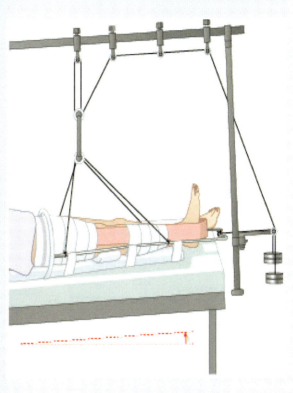

Chapter 10

Chapter 10: Elective Orthopaedics

Common Elective Procedures and Post-Op Complications

Written by Jimmy Ng

Chapter 10: Elective Orthopaedics Contents

1. Total hip replacement — p139
2. Total knee replacement — p142
3. Arthroscopy — p143
4. Post-Op: acute kidney injury — p144
5. Post-Op: hyponatremia — p146

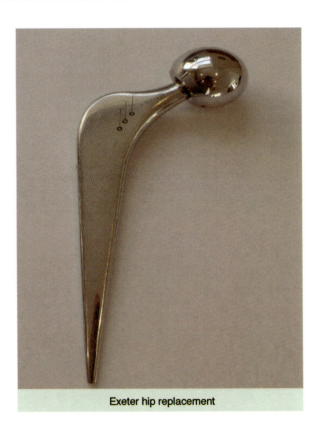

Exeter hip replacement

Elective Ward Round Assessment Checklist

History: Pre-op State

Past medical history	• Medical conditions • Medications • Anti-coagulant therapy • Reason for anti-coagulation • Upper arm • Shoulder / clavicle • Other ....
VTE assessment	• Anticoagulant prescribed and mobilisation
Social history	• Pre-op mobility • Alcohol • Home situation • Who is at home with them? • Do they have stairs?

Post-op State

Pain	• Pain?
Associated symptoms	• Nausea • Constipation • Passing urine
Current mobility	• Chair • Frame • 2 sticks • Stairs

Chapter 10

	Examination
Observation	• Observations • Wounds • Drain volumes • Calves
Hip Replacement	• Leg length • Sciatic nerve (ankle dorsiflexion) • Femoral artery (dorsalis pedis / popliteal pulse)
Knee replacement	• Range of movement • Common peroneal nerve (ankle dorsiflexion) • Popliteal artery (dorsalis pedis / posterior tibial pulse)
Upper limb joint replacement	• Axillary nerve power and sensation • Median nerve power and sensation • Ulna nerve power and sensation • Radial nerve power and sensation

	Day 1 Jobs
Bloods	• FBC, U+Es, INR*
X-ray Mobilise	• As per post op instructions - *if anticoagulation planned

3 Topics Not To Miss
1. Dislocated hip   3. Occluded artery 2. Drop foot

ELECTIVE

Elective orthopaedics provides a different challenge to trauma patients. These patients should be well prior to their procedure and should have passed through various pre-assessment hurdles before being admitted. Most will be admitted on the day of surgery so you will not see them until their operation has been completed. Some units have protocols requiring you to complete drug charts and venous thromboprophylaxis assessment in the admission lounge, and this saves you and the poor soul who is on call from doing it when the patient returns to the ward, invariably late in the afternoon.

There is a wide range of elective procedures which are beyond the scope of the book. The bread and butter procedures, hip and knee replacements and arthroscopies are covered, as well as the management of the more common metabolic complications that you will need to manage.

1. Total hip replacement

Indications

Any conditions which cause degeneration and pain in the hip joint are indications for total hip replacement (THR). THR will be considered when conservative measures have failed. Some of the most common conditions include osteoarthritis, inflammatory arthritis and avascular necrosis. THR is also a treatment option for trauma to the hip joint, such as intracapsular fracture of the proximal femur.

Types of total hip replacement

THR as its name suggests, consists of replacement of both the acetabulum and femur components of the hip joint. There are a lot of different THR implants available. Their use depends on surgeon's preference and the implant's safety profile.

In general terms, they can be cemented, uncemented or hybrid. Cemented THR has cemented femoral and acetabulum components, whereas in uncemented THR, both components are uncemented.

A hybrid THR is when the femoral stem component is cemented but the acetabulum is uncemented.

Post-operative care

As a junior doctor on the orthopaedic wards, one should always check the operation notes for specific post-operative instructions. Routine post-operative care includes prophylactic antibiotics, weight bearing status (usually full weight bearing, unless stated otherwise), full blood count, urea and electrolytes, post-operative pelvic x ray and thromboprophylaxis.

Although THR is one of the most successful orthopaedic operations, complications can occur either immediately or at a later stage.

Dislocation

Dislocation is the most serious mechanical complication of THR. Patients usually have an abduction wedge or pillow placed in between their legs post-operatively to keep leg in abduction so that it stays in joint. Dislocation can be identified by leg length discrepancy, significant hip pain and neurovascular compromise.

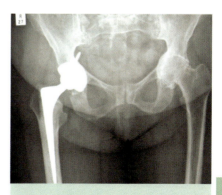

Figure 10.1 AP both hips with a hybrid (cemented stem and uncemented cup) in situ.

An urgent x ray must be requested and the orthopaedic registrar informed. A dislocated THR needs to be reduced under general anaesthesia as soon as possible. Reduction needs to be completed as an emergency if there is any evidence of neurovascular compromise, such as a foot drop. For the first dislocation, a reduction should be performed in theatre as it allows for a thorough assessment of stability. Recurrent dislocations may be reduced in the Emergency Department.

Fracture

Fracture is uncommon during total hip replacement but can happen especially during uncemented femoral stem placement. This is usually identified intraoperatively and dealt with immediately. However, if a fracture which is not known previously is identified on the post-operative x ray, you should keep the patient on bedrest until reviewed by the orthopaedic registrar.

Foot drop

Foot drop is a sign of damage to the sciatic nerve. This is often traction injury, but can also be a presentation of dislocation as the femoral head compresses on the sciatic nerve.

Pelvic bleeding

Pelvic bleeding is a rare complication of total hip replacement. This can happen when augmentation screws are used to secure the acetabular component. Patients with pelvic bleeding will present with haemorrhagic shock, tachycardia and persistently dropping haemoglobin. An urgent CT angiogram with possible embolization will be required.

Venous thromboembolism

Patients undergoing lower limb arthroplasty are at increased risk of venous thromboembolism including deep vein thrombosis and pulmonary embolus. All patients should have thromboprophylaxis according to the local hospital policy.

Infection

Infection is a major concern in any orthopaedic procedure, especially arthroplasty. All patients undergoing orthopaedic surgery using a prosthesis will require antibiotics prophylaxis according to your local hospital policy. Any patients with suspected sepsis during the post-operative period should have their surgical wound inspected.

DAILY ASSESSMENT OF POST-OPERATIVE TOTAL HIP REPLACEMENT

- Complete assessment checklist
- Check operative note for mobilisation strategy and post-op plan
- Check venousthromboprophylaxis has been prescribed
- Check wound – can check if dressing is dry unless there is a concern about profuse bleeding (keeps the wound as clear as possible)
- Consider discharge planning (often day 4-5)
- Confirm post-op follow up arrangements

ONGOING ADMISSION REQUIRED UNTIL

- Patient mobile and has "passed" physio & OT
- Wound dry
- X-ray satisfactory
- Blood tests and observations normal

Elective Orthopaedics: Total Hip Replacement

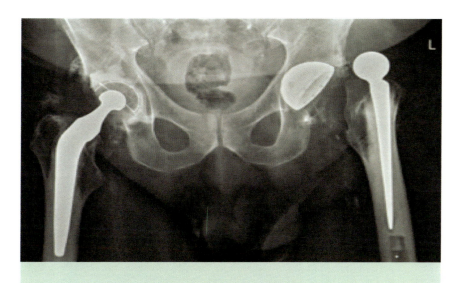

Figure 10.2 Dislocated left total hip replacement

ORTHOPAEDIC EMERGENCY: TIME TO WAKE UP THE REGISTRAR

- Suspected dislocation: organise an x-ray and call the registrar
- Fracture on x-ray: put patient on bed rest and inform registrar during daylight hours
- Foot drop: document findings, organise x-ray if hip painful and inform registrar during daylight hours

2. Total knee replacement

Indications

1. Osteoarthritis
2. Inflammatory arthritis
3. Trauma

Types of total knee replacement

Similar to hip replacement, total knee replacement (TKR) can be classified into cemented, uncemented and hybrid. In patients with a single compartment disease/arthritis, they may be eligible for an unicompartmental knee replacement if they meet the specific criteria.

Potential complications

Similar complications can occur in knee replacements as in hip replacements. These complications include infection, venous thromboembolism and fracture. There are also other complications specific to knee replacements.

Neurovascular injury

The neurovascular bundle lies closely to the posterior knee capsule and is at risk of injury during tibial cuts and retractor placement. Neurovascular status of the leg can be easily examined by feeling for peripheral pulses, capillary refill, ankle dorsiflexion and sensation in the first dorsal web space.

Another structure at risk is the common peroneal nerve. This nerve lies in the posterolateral aspect of the knee and travels around the fibular head. Correction of knee deformity through knee replacement can put the nerve under stretch, resulting in nerve palsy and foot drop. The most common deformity to cause nerve palsy is valgus flexion deformity. In the first instance, all compression bandages should be released and knee placed in flexion. After that, the orthopaedic registrar must be informed.

Post-operative care

Routine post-operative care includes post-operative x ray, blood tests, physiotherapy, weight bearing status (normally full weight bearing), removal of drain after 24 hours (if used) and antibiotics prophylaxis.

DAILY ASSESSMENT OF POST-OPERATIVE TOTAL KNEE REPLACEMENT

- Complete assessment checklist
- Check operative note for mobilisation strategy and post-op plan
- Check venousthromboprophylaxis has been prescribed
- Check wound – can check if dressing is dry unless there is a concern about profuse bleeding (keeps the wound as clear as possible)
- Consider discharge planning (often day 4-5)
- Confirm post-op follow up arrangements

ONGOING ADMISSION REQUIRED UNTIL

- Patient mobile and has "passed" physio & OT
- Wound dry
- X-ray satisfactory
- Blood tests and observations normal

ORTHOPAEDIC EMERGENCY: TIME TO WAKE UP THE REGISTRAR

- Fracture on x-ray: put patient on bed rest and inform registrar during daylight hours
- Foot drop: document findings, organise x-ray if knee painful and inform registrar during daylight hours

3. Arthroscopy

Arthroscopic surgery is keyhole surgery for bones and joints. It uses one or more access portals to allow positioning of a camera inside the joint. The joint is then distended with fluid to give space to work with various tools such as nibblers, graspers and special arthroscopic tools such as suture passers, shavers and diathermy cutters.

Arthroscopic surgery is very effective for soft tissue injuries where minimal tissue trauma is required. Soft tissue defects can be managed in situ without the need for massive exposure. Recovery is often faster and rehabilitation begun sooner.

However, there is a caution. There are several studies that demonstrate that arthroscopic debridement and washout of the knee is not effective when done for degenerate tears to the menisci. This is a controversial topic, with vast deviations in practice within the U.K. and around the world. The accepted bottom line is that arthroscopic debridement is effective in fresh traumatic tears (especially in the young) and will improve mechanical symptoms of locking and giving way. It is unlikely to improve, and may even exacerbate, pain from arthritis.

Common sites for arthroscopy and indications:

SHOULDER	• Diagnostic arthroscopy • Rotator cuff tear • Subacromial decompression • Sepsis
ANKLE	• Diagnostic arthroscopy • Osteochondral defects • Removal of loose bodies • Sepsis
ELBOW	• Diagnostic arthroscopy • Removal of loose bodies • Arthrolysis
KNEE	• Diagnostic arthroscopy • Meniscal tear • Cruciate ligament injury • Osteochondral defects • Removal of loose bodies • Sepsis
WRIST	• Diagnostic • Triangular fibrocartilage complex tear • Chondral lesions

Chapter 10

Post-operative care

Post-operative care is dependent on the pathology. Early mobilisation should be encouraged and patients are normally discharged on the day of surgery.

DAILY ASSESSMENT OF POST-OPERATIVE ARTHROSCOPY

- Complete assessment checklist
- Check operative note for mobilisation strategy and post-op plan
- Consider discharge planning

ONGOING ADMISSION REQUIRED UNTIL

- Patient mobile and has "passed" physio & OT
- Wound dry

ORTHOPAEDIC EMERGENCY: TIME TO WAKE UP THE REGISTRAR

- Compartment syndrome – exceptionally rare complication of knee arthroscopy due to pressurised infiltration of fluid into the joint

4. Post-Op: Acute Kidney Injury

Acute kidney injury (AKI) is an acute deterioration of renal function, based on creatinine levels and urine output. 1 in 5 emergency admissions have acute kidney injury and those in hospital with AKI have a mortality rate of 23.6%. AKI is common among orthopaedic patients, particularly the elderly. As a junior doctor on the orthopaedic ward, one must be able to identify those at risk, diagnose AKI early and manage the condition promptly.

Patients at risk of AKI

- Elderly patients
- Intraoperative blood loss
- Chronic kidney disease
- Diabetes
- Heart failure

CAUSES OF AKI

- **Prerenal:**
  Hypovolaemia
  Bleeding
  ACE inhibitors and angiotensin receptor blockers
  NSAIDS

- **Renal:**
  Nephrotoxic agent such as contrast agent
  Glomerulonephritis

- **Postrenal:**
  Calculi
  Malignancy
  Pelvic mass

ELECTIVE

Diagnosis of AKI

NICE recommended using (p)RIFLE, AKIN or KDIGO criteria to diagnose and detect acute kidney injury:

- Increase in serum creatinine of ≥26 micromol/litre within 48 hours
- ≥50% rise in serum creatinine within the last 7 days
- urine output of less than 0.5 ml/kg/hour for more than 6 hours

Management of AKI

Initial management of patients with AKI should include a thorough clinical examination, review of notes including operation note and drug card. Urinalysis should be completed as well as urinary catheterisation if severe. Clinical examination must be undertaken to assess fluid status, examine wound site and drain volume to ensure no ongoing blood loss.

Management of AKI depends on the underlying pathology. There are prerenal, renal and postrenal causes of AKI. In elective orthopaedic patients, the most common reason for AKI is hypovolaemia due to intraoperative blood loss and intravascular volume depletion.

ASSESSMENT OF ACUTE KIDNEY INJURY IN ELECTIVE PATIENTS

- Assess fluid status
- Urinary catheterisation (if required)
- Urinalysis
- IV fluids if hypovolaemic
- Stop al nephrotoxic drugs
- Treat underlying pathology
- Ultrasound scan (if no response to initial management)
- Seek medical advice if no response

ONGOING ADMISSION REQUIRED UNTIL

- U&Es improved

ORTHOPAEDIC EMERGENCY: TIME TO WAKE UP THE REGISTRAR

- Life-threatening acidosis or hyperkalaemia – though may be worth calling renal or medical registrar first!

5. Post-Op: Hyponatraemia

Hyponatraemia is defined as sodium level of less than 135 mmol/L. This is a very common electrolyte abnormality but is often overlooked. Orthopaedic patients are particularly at risk, especially the elderly due to other comorbidities and concurrent medication use.

Untreated hyponatraemia can lead to cerebral oedema and coma. It is therefore vital that this condition is diagnosed and treated promptly.

Early clinical features of hyponatraemia include anorexia, nausea and lethargy. Late signs such as disorientation, agitation, seizure and coma indicate cerebral oedema which requires rapid correction with hypertonic saline and close monitoring.

Diagnostic and management approach

It is not within the scope of this book to discuss the full management of hyponatraemia. This chapter aims to outline a recommended management approach. The management of hyponatraemia depends on the fluid status and presence of symptoms.

Asymptomatic

In asymptomatic patients, their electrolyte levels should be monitored closely (at least daily). In those who are hypovolaemic, intravenous infusion of normal saline will inhibit antidiuretic hormone secretion and facilitate correction of the sodium level. In those who are euvolaemic or hypervolaemic, a fluid restriction regime (<1L/day) should be used.

The medications should be reviewed and all hypotonic fluid therapy stopped.

Symptomatic

In patients with significant symptoms secondary to hyponatraemia (such as seizure and reduced consciousness), they need rapid correction of their serum sodium by the means of hypertonic saline. Advice from the medical team should be sought urgently before commencing this treatment.

ASSESSMENT OF HYPONATRIMIA IN ELECTIVE PATIENTS

- Calculate severity and identify if patient symptomatic
- Review medications
- Request daily bloods and paired urinary and serum osmolarities
- If severe hyponatrimia refer to medics or endoctine team
- If patient hypovolaemic then fluid restrict, if dry then rehydrate

ONGOING ADMISSION REQUIRED UNTIL

- Sodium level improved

ORTHOPAEDIC EMERGENCY: TIME TO WAKE UP THE REGISTRAR

- Seizures – may be worth calling the medical registrar first!

Further reading

- 1. Verbalis JG, Goldsmith SR, Greenberg A, Korzelius C, Schrier RW, Sterns RH, et al. Diagnosis, Evaluation, and Treatment of Hyponatremia: Expert Panel Recommendations. The American Journal of Medicine. 2013 Oct 1;126(10):S1–42.

- 2. Miller MD, Thompson SR, Hart JA. Review of Orthopaedics. 6th Edition. Philadelphia: Elsevier; 2012.

- 3. Learmonth ID, Young C, Rorabeck C. The operation of the century: total hip replacement. The Lancet. 2007 Nov 2;370(9597):1508–19.

Chapter 11: Next Steps

How To Become A Trauma And Orthopaedic Surgeon

Chapter 11: Next Steps Contents

1. Training scheme overview	p148	4. Audit ideas	p154
2. Work-based assessment	p150	5. Interviews	p156
3. Courses and qualificatiosn	p154		

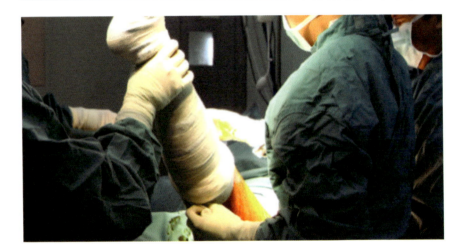

So, you have made it to the end of this book. Congratulations, and I hope with your clinical experience that you have gained in Orthopaedics you have been inspired to take your training further.

This chapter will review the entry requirements for Trauma and Orthopaedics in the United Kingdom and make suggestions to help best position yourself to gain a training job in this speciality.

1. Training scheme overview

There are several routes through to the endpoint of a consultant post. The most structured is to gain entry onto the training program at CT1 (postgraduate year 3). This will involve at least 2 years of core surgical training and then competitive entry into the ST3 (registrar, postgraduate year 5+) program. This leads to a Certificate of completion of training (CCT) and eligibility to apply for consultant posts.

Next Steps: Training Scheme Overview

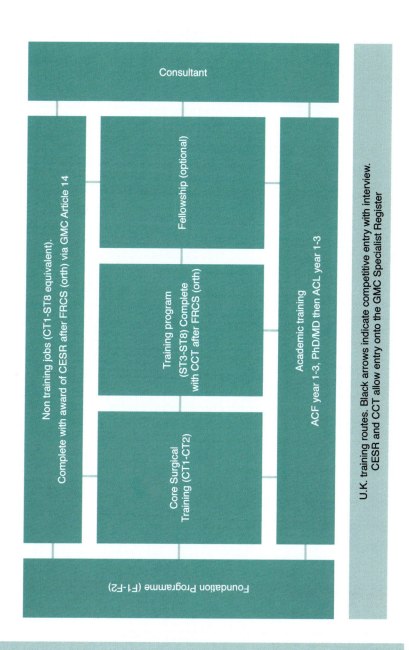

Figure 11.1 UK training pathway

Chapter 11

Alternatively, there are a multitude of non-training jobs available that you can undertake. You will gain experience in these posts and still have the opportunity to rotate through different sub-specialities. However, beware –if you choose this route then you will be responsible for documenting all your own training and preparing a portfolio for presentation to gain a Certificate of Eligibility for Specialist Registration (CESR). This is hard work, and the level of evidence required is high and very time consuming if started at the end of your training. If you are thinking of taking this alternative route then start preparing evidence for your portfolio early.

Getting into core surgical training and registrar training

The requirements for core surgical training and ST3 training are available online. They are available on the speciality training website (http://specialtytraining.hee.nhs.uk/) and are worth finding and reading.

The key requirements that are in the 2016 person specification are summarised in the table on the next page. These highlighted requirements are summarised from the person specifications for the 2015 intake, and the full specification is available at the speciality training website. These requirements can be met with evidence from work-based assessments, portfolio evidence and research and audit projects as well as performance at interview.

2. Work-based assessments

As a foundation trainee, you are expected to complete a number of work-based assessments every year. This may feel like a vast number of assessments, with a struggle to track down core trainees, registrars and consultants to get the things finished and they do feel like a tick box exercise. However, the best work based assessments demonstrate improvement and can be used as an effective weapon in your next interview if you can show you have completed a learning cycle.

For trainees not in the foundation scheme, paper versions of the work-based assessments and instructions for their use are available at the JCST website (www.iscp.ac.uk)

To complete a learning cycle following a work-based assessment first reflect on what has been said in the assessment and document (either on the assessment or elsewhere) a summary of this reflection. Next, identify one or two weaknesses in your practice and identify a specific solution, such as completing an e-learning module or performing a set number of procedures. Once you have done these actions then repeat an observed practice and complete a follow up work-based assessment to document your improvement. A summary of the learning cycle is a powerful tool to include in your portfolio as evidence of:

1. Reflective practice
2. Values
3. Clinical skills
4. Organisation
5. Commitment to speciality

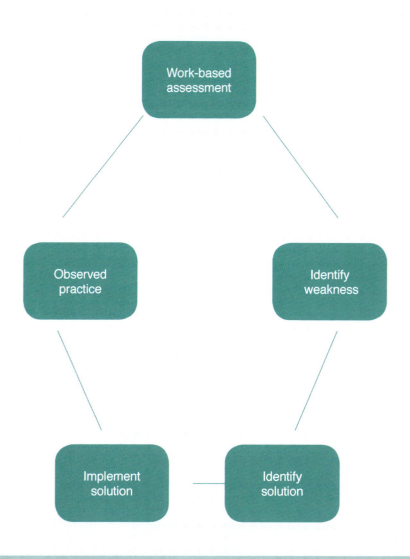

Figure 11.2 Learning cycle based around work-based assessment

Chapter 11

Requirement	Core Surgical Entry (CT1)	Registrar (ST3)
• Eligibility: qualifications	• Medical degree • Advance life support (ALS) • Degree from UK medical school or IELTS score of 7.0 in each domain and overall score of 7.5	• Medical degree • MRCS • ATLS • CCrISP • Basic course on fracture management • Basic surgical skills course • Casting techniques course • Degree from UK medical school or IELTS score of 7.0 in each domain and overall score of 7.5
• Eligibility: experience	• Currently in foundation programme or • 12 months experience following full GMC registration and certificate of achievement of foundation competencies • 18 months experience or less in surgery	• Completion of CT1 competencies on ISCP by time of application and evidence of CT2 competencies by time of appointment. • At least 24 months experience in surgery (excluding foundation programme) with at least 10 months in trauma

Next Steps: ST3 T&O Selection Criteria

• Clinical skills	• Work based assessments in and examples of knowledge, problem solving, prioritisation, initial management of unwell patient and visuospatial skills	• Work based assessments in and examples of knowledge, problem solving, prioritisation, initial management of unwell patient and visuospatial skills • Validated logbook
• Research and audit	• Evidence of research projects and degrees, presentations, publications and teaching	• Evidence of research projects and degrees, presentations, publications and teaching
• Personal skills	• Communication skills • Problem solving • Empathy • Management • Team working • Organisation • IT • Vigilance • Situational awareness • Coping with pressure • Values • Outside interests	• Communication skills • Problem solving • Management • Teamwork • Organisation • Vigilance • Situational awareness • Coping with pressure • Values
• Commitment to speciality	• Initiative and enthusiasm • Demonstrable interest • Attendance at teaching • Self-reflective practice • Evidence of extra activities	• Realistic insight • Knowledge of training programme • Insight into capacity and importance of feedback • Evidence of career plan

CAREERS

153

Chapter 11

3. Courses and qualifications

Essential courses (ATLS, CCrISP and Basic Surgical Skills) that are run in conjunction with the Royal College of surgeons are advertised on the Royal College website. These are well worth booking early and completing, as it has been known for courses to be cancelled last minute resulting in individuals becoming ineligible to apply for jobs.

The most recognised course on fracture management is the AO principles course. This is a 4 day course and is very comprehensive with skills in surgical planning, sawbone fixation and operative technique. However, it is very expensive. Dates for this course are advertised on the AO website . If budget isn't a worry then consider taking the course in Davos, Switzerland (AO headquarters) where the teaching is interspersed with skiing and apres-ski!

The addition of casting courses is a relatively recent inclusion and it is unclear as to the expected level or duration of the course. The Royal National Orthopaedics Hospital (Stanmore, London) host a good 1 day course . Alternatively, many local courses have now been established. Contact your local deanery to see if there is one in your area.

TOP TIPS
1. Complete courses early
2. Plan to spread the cost between FY2 and CT1 and the early portion of CT2
3. Some of the courses will help with MRCS revision, especially CCrISP and ATLS

4. Audit and research

Research skills are difficult to obtain. Speak to your consultant early as research takes time. If you don't have much research yet then don't worry too much. A recent survey of successful ST3 candidates discovered that the majority of candidates did not have any publications and only a handful of presentations. Instead it is better to focus your time on MRCS, interview practice and completing some closed loop audits.

An audit is an evaluation of current practice, audited against a set standard. Audits need to be relevant, identify something that can be changed and improved and also achievable. Aim to complete at least 1 per year, ideally within your 4 month rotation. Present these at your local audit meeting, and submit an abstract to larger meetings to gain full credit for your work. Below are a set of audit ideas that can be easily achieved during a four month rotation.

Management of open fractures:

Standards: BOA Boast 4 guidelines

IV antibiotics within 3 hours of injury

Documentation of neurovascular status
Debridement within 24h
Definitive stabilisation and soft tissue cover within 72h

Design: Retrospective looking at ED cards coded as open fracture

Intervention: Education and poster for use in ED

Timeframe: Initial data collection will take 2-3 afternoons. Re-audit in 1 month following intervention

Documentation of neurovascular status in paediatric supracondylar fractures:

Standards: BOA Boast 11 guidelines

Next Steps: Audit and Research

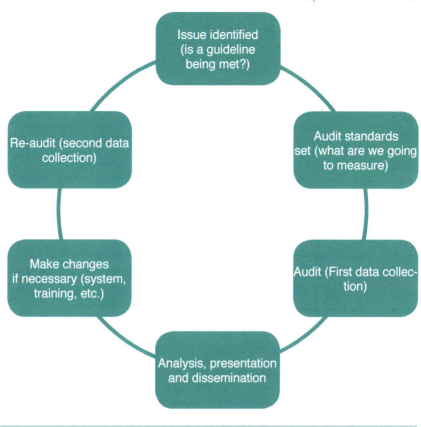

Figure 11.3 Audit cycle

Documentation of radial pulse and capillary refill time (CRT)
Documentation of radial, median (including anterior interosseous) and ulna nerve
Time to theatre
Design: Retrospective looking at theatre records and ED cards

Intervention: Proforma or aide-memoire for T&O SHOs

Timeframe: Initial data collection will take 2-3 afternoons. Re-audit in 1 month following intervention

Timings of prophylaxic antibiotics for joint replacement

Standards: AAOS guidelines or local policy
Antibiotic within 1h of incision
Antibiotic choice as per local guideline
Antibiotic discontinued after 24h
Antibiotic given at what times post-op

Design: can be retrospective by pulling drug cards or prospective looking at all the joint replacements over a 5 day period

Intervention: Sticker or change in documentation

Timeframe: Prospective data collection may

be quicker and prevent the need for pulling notes. Re-audit 1 month after intervention

Analgesia following hip fracture

Standards: NICE guideline CG 124
Pain assessment on arrival to hospital
Pain assessment within 30 mins of initial analgesia
Hourly pain assessments until pain settled
Regular pain assessment with observations

Design: retrospective review of nursing documentation as patients are admitted with fractures

Intervention: Pain scores on observation chart or promote alternative analgesics such as fascia iliaca blocks

Timeframe 1-2 weeks to collect data

Acute kidney injury in post-operative orthopaedic patients

Standards: NICE guidelines CG169
Documentation of cause of AKI
Documentation of medications review
Documanetation of urine dipstick result
Daily bloods
Medical (renal) review for patients with grade 3 AKI or need for dialysis

Design: retrospective review of casenotes

Intervention: Sticker or proforma

Timeframe: 1-2 weeks to collect data from case notes.

TOP TIPS

1. Aim to complete a minimum of 1 audit per year
2. Present your findings and obtain feedback
3. Re-audit following intervention and identify effect

---

5. Interview practice

Over the next few years, preparing for exams and interviews will become part of your day to day life if you choose to go into orthopaedics. The first hurdle is the Core Surgical Training interview. This is a standardised interview to test you have a reasonable grasp of English, understand how to manage sick patients and confirm that you have done some surgical rotations. You are applying for the entry level jobs so it is a reasonable prospect of getting a job. However, you will need a decent portfolio and some interview questions prepared to get a better chance of the top jobs in the deanery you want.

Recently, the surgical recruitment for core surgery has included a checklist for sections required in your portfolio. When I interviewed, I had approximately 10 pages for each section, ensuring that each of the domains in the person specification was covered. Keep it to 1 folder, more is too much and won't be read and may even lose you marks. Previous sections included:

1. Medical qualifications
2. CPD courses
3. Exceptional performance in undergraduate / foundation years
4. Clinical / procedural experience
5. Clinical audit / service improvement
6. Teaching
7. Presentations / abstracts / publications
8. Research
9. Leadership and teamwork
10. Commitment to surgery

The time taken to prepare this portfolio is quite surprising. Plan to have the portfolio ready by Christmas in your FY2 year to leave a couple of months to prepare for the interview. Most invest in a swanky folder to keep this in. This can't do any harm, and you want to give the best possible

Next Steps: Interview Practice

first impression to keep up and potentially overtake the other applicants.

The ST3 interview is very similar to the core surgical interview in format, but a new level in intensity and competition. The stations will test anatomy, clinical knowledge, commitment to surgery via portfolio, topical orthopaedic knowledge and communication and practical skills. Expect the unexpected; my cohort thought there would be no chance of being tested on endoscopic skills only to be presented with a laparoscopic trainer. Again, have your portfolio prepared early, do practice questions with other core surgical trainees and subject yourself to grilling by consultants in the trauma meetings and in theatre.

Interview courses and preparation

These represent a great investment to build experience and identify weaknesses in your interview technique. Core Surgery Interview (www.coresurgeryinterview.com) offers courses, books and an online questions bank for core surgery applicnats and is widely used by the majority of applicants. The Royal Society of Medicine runs a great 1 day course called speciality application series: core surgical training. This gives good hints and tips and gives you an idea as to what the competition is likely to be.

For ST3, several courses are available. Orthointerview (www.orthointerview.com) runs an excellent course which is split into knowledge lectures and practice question sessions. This spans two days in Bristol and is well worth considering. They also offer a question bank of interview questions to help you prepare.

> **TOP TIPS**
> 1. Prepare your portfolio early
> 2. Do plenty of interview practice
> 3. Good luck!

References

1. https://www.rcseng.ac.uk/courses/course-search/regional-courses/regional-search

2. https://aotrauma.aofoundation.org

3. https://www.rnoh.nhs.uk/health-professionals/courses-conferences

4. https://www.boa.ac.uk/wp-content/uploads/2014/12/BOAST-4.pdf

5. https://www.boa.ac.uk/wp-content/uploads/2014/12/BOAST-11.pdf

6. http://www.aaos.org/about/papers/advistmt/1027.asp

7. https://www.nice.org.uk/guidance/cg124/chapter/1-Guidance

8. https://www.nice.org.uk/guidance/cg169

9. https://www.rsm.ac.uk/events/events-listing/2015-2016/sections/trainees-committee/trg06-specialty-application-series-core-surgical-training.aspx

10. https://www.orthointerview.com/

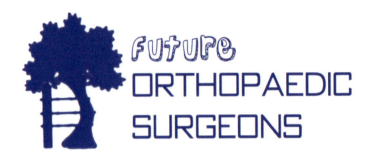

www.futureorthopaedicsurgeons.com

JOIN ONLINE NOW

 Interested in Trauma and Orthopaedic Surgery?

Future Orthopaedic Surgeons is the only international society for medical students and early-years doctors who are passionate about pursuing a career in the popular field of trauma and orthopaedic surgery.

FOS membership inlcudes access to the Journal of Undergraduate Trauma and Orthopaedics (JUTO), career resources and prizes to help improve your CV ahead of applications. FOS members also get the latest updates and information regarding Trauma and Orthopaedic Surgery.

Printed in Great Britain
by Amazon